Rise Up

with the

Hope of

Healing

My Journey toward Spiritual,
Physical, and Mental Well-Being

Sam Crow

RISE UP WITH THE HOPE OF HEALING
Copyright © 2020 by Sam Crow

This material is not intended as a substitution for medical advice. Please consult a physician before undertaking any changes to diet, exercise, or medication.

Plexus Worldwide does not claim to treat or cure any disease—rather, it offers hope for people to live a life of health and happiness.

Unless otherwise noted, scripture quotations are taken from *the Holy Bible, New Living Translation*, copyright ©1996, 2004, 2007 by Tyndale House Foundation. Used by permission of Tyndale House Publishers, Inc., Carol Stream, Illinois 60188. All rights reserved. Scripture marked AMPC taken from the Amplified® Bible, Classic Edition, Copyright © 1954, 1958, 1962, 1964, 1965, 1987 by The Lockman Foundation. Used by permission. Scripture marked NIV taken from The Holy Bible, New International Version®, NIV® Copyright ©1973, 1978, 1984, 2011 by Biblica, Inc.® Used by permission. All rights reserved worldwide.

Printed in Canada

Print ISBN: 978-1-4866-2011-1
eBook ISBN: 978-1-4866-2012-8

Word Alive Press
119 De Baets Street, Winnipeg, MB R2J 3R9
www.wordalivepress.ca

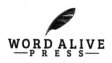 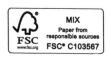

Cataloguing in Publication may be obtained through Library and Archives Canada

Dedication

First, I give thanks to Jesus for His gift of life and His love. I could have never made this journey without Him by my side every day. He is the one and only great Healer of the Universe.

I want to thank my family. To my husband Ted, for your everlasting love and faith in me as we follow God's plan for our lives. To my daughter Ashley, for your unconditional love and forgiveness as I learn and grow every day. I love you both so very dearly.

I dedicate this book to my dear friend Kathy. During our innumerable visits, you have encouraged me to share what I have learned through my journey to healing. I hope you always know how much I treasure our friendship. Some friendships are only for a season, but ours is one for Eternity.

Finally, I want to thank God for the miracle that came through His children, making this book possible.

Contents

Acknowledgements

I would like to thank all those at Word Alive Press for the beautiful experience I had with them as they shared their gifts. Thanks to Jen Jandavs-Hedlin, publisher, for your many phone calls, encouragement, and honesty. I am so very thankful I met you. To Marina Reis, project manager: thank you for your patience and many e-mails back and forth as you guided me through the many decisions I needed to make. I am truly thankful for all your help. Thanks to Matthew Knight for doing the final edit of my work to make sure it was the best it could be. I am so very grateful for your patience with me in the world of technology. You went above and beyond for me, and I will always be so thankful for your kindness. To the person with whom I shared my thoughts for the cover and the design (even though I never met you)—you made it became a reality. Thank you. If you need a Canadian publishing company, I would highly recommend this one. It was a wonderful journey!

Introduction

Life is hard here on earth. Over years of listening to the pain of so many people around me, the desire was placed in my heart to share what my life experiences have taught me. I believe many people are struggling in a world that has completely lost its balance with life. When our lives go out of balance, it opens the door to disease in the body, as well as creating an environment for many emotional, mental, and spiritual illnesses.

When I began to have health issues back in 2009, I could never have imagined the real journey that this would take me on—not until I was brought down to my knees in 2013 when Lyme disease came knocking on my door. It's amazing how life works in your time of need. I eventually learned the road I was going down could be a wonderful teacher if only I would open my heart to receive the healing I needed. Through my journey of physical illness, I began to learn that what I needed was deeper spiritual healing.

Once I allowed the Holy Spirit to show me the areas of my life that I needed to heal from, then the true healing began. When you heal on the inside first, it allows greater healing in your physical, emotional, and mental being. In the end, this complete healing brought me to a much better place—one I believe we can all find.

I give thanks to God, because He has never given up on me. As time goes by and I pause now to reflect, I realize my journey is truly about knowing who I am in Christ. This journey is one I will always appreciate, as I believe God has brought me through many challenges for a greater purpose. The very pain of these experiences has set me free. As I always say, "Freedom begins with honesty." If you are not honest with yourself, how can you ever truly be set free? Now my desire is to share my experiences with others, so they, too, can see Jesus and His amazing love. I am truly thankful He has given me the gift of time to study, learn, and write this book.

As we take this journey together, you will personally come to know how dearly you are loved, and that you are never alone. You are a child of God and He loves you just the way you are. Come walk with us as you begin your own journey, and allow yourself to receive freely what God so desperately wants to give you: a new life and everlasting healing.

Let the healing begin...

"I will give you back your health and heal your wounds," says the Lord.

—Jeremiah 30:17

Then I heard the Lord asking, "Whom should I send as a messenger to this people? Who will go for us?" I said, "Here I am. Send me."
—Isaiah 6:8

The Alarm of My Heart
Chapter One

As I looked in the rear-view mirror, my heart began to race. The flashing red lights sent my heart into panic mode. What was I doing? If only I hadn't pulled over to grab the lighter that had fallen to the floor, I wouldn't be in this mess.

As the officer tapped on my window, the tears fell even harder. This was the stage of my confession. "Why did you pull over?" he asked.

My answer was simple. I tried to explain my tears and the struggle of wanting a cigarette after the news I had heard about my step-grandmother. She had been diagnosed with cancer, and I was really upset. Fear began to sink in as he asked for my registration and licence, but the question he asked next was even more frightening. "Have you been drinking?"

With his questioning came honesty from my heart. I had to tell the truth. Yes, I'd had a few beers, and now this was the consequence for my decision. I was extremely blessed that night. When the officer learned how close to home I was, he sent me on my way. His words struck me to the core of my soul: "Don't you ever drink and drive again." That was my warning signal, and thank God I listened to him.

Now twenty-three years later, how was this possible? I had made another bad choice, but the truth would set me free.

It was May 22, 2011, when I woke up at our cottage with a hangover. When I went downstairs, I was shocked to find I had drunk two bottles of wine the night before. Things had to change! I knew today was going to be different—but why? I believe it was because I asked a question, which meant my heart was ready to receive an answer.

I went down to the lake and stood there, then looked up and asked, "Why do I keep making the same mistakes and hurting the people I love?" As I was pondering that question, I started remembering the things I had said and done. I fell to my knees in shame. The very thing I complained about others doing, I had just done myself. I had gotten in the vehicle drunk and driven to the store.

How many times in our lives do we judge others? If we are willing to look in the mirror at our own life, we will begin to see ourselves for who we truly are. We sometimes recognize things in other people so easily because we have the same qualities. That day made me realize how different my story could have gone. I could have killed someone or myself, I could have ended up in jail, or I could have caused a financial burden to my family by writing off the vehicle. That was the day the alarm went off in my heart!

I went up to the cottage and I got my Bible out. I randomly opened it to Ephesians and these words jumped off the page: *"Don't be drunk with wine, because that will ruin your life. Instead, be filled with the Holy Spirit..."* (Ephesians 5:18). That was a life-changing day for me. I got dressed and went to church at Harvest in Muskoka. It was as if the message was written just for me. It was called "An Invitation to God," based on Isaiah 55. I cried during the whole service, and the pastor left us with two questions to ponder: "Do you want a different life? Are you tired of how you are living?"

My answer was yes—I was tired and ready for a change. My usual routine was to stop by the local grocery store and get a bottle of red wine for my afternoon on the dock. But that day the small, quiet voice said, "You don't need that anymore. I am with you."

When I got back to the cottage, I was excited to share what had happened to me that morning. But I would quickly learn that this was not the day to share about the new life I was beginning. When I tried to apologize to my family for my behaviour the night before, they didn't want to listen to me. Why would they believe me after I had been drunk so many times? I knew it was time to stop talking and show them with actions that my life had been changed.

After that day at the cottage, I would love to say that everything instantly changed—but I can't. Was it easy? No, it was hard work, and I could never have done it in my own strength. I needed God's help. A scripture that I would repeat to myself constantly was *"For I can do everything through Christ, who gives me strength"* (Philippians 4:13). Anytime something went wrong or I got into a serious discussion with my family, it seemed they would inevitably bring up my drinking days, even though it had been many years since I had drank. I would get so frustrated and wonder, *What's the use? I may as well drink because they don't believe I've changed.* But I heard the Lord say to me, "Just keep going, Sam; it's just going to take a bit more time for them to see this new you is here to stay."

What's your story? What are you going through right now that has brought you down to your knees?

Is it the loss of someone you love, or perhaps an illness knocking on your door or that of a loved one? Could it be an addiction to another choice? Drugs, cigarettes, food, people-pleasing, pornography, gambling, hoarding—or do depression and anxiety have a hold on you? Have you just lost your job, or are struggling with your finances because of something out of your control? Are you trying to stay afloat but don't know how to cope with the battles of everyday life?

I believe many people don't realize the power they can have over their lives just by learning to control their thoughts. When we learn how to control this, it instantly starts to create more healing. The more you focus on the positive things in your life, the better it gets. The mind truly is the battlefield where what we think about becomes the enemy in our own lives if we are not careful to focus on the good things. What a person feels to be true in their heart is what they begin to believe as the truth.

So how do you retrain the mind? It takes a lot of hard work, and with practice, it will become second nature to you. When a negative thought comes in, kick it out right away with something positive—with an outcome you hope to see happen in your life. There are many times when I find singing a favourite worship song to myself will quickly stop any negative thinking. I love the chorus to a song that I often sing to myself: "Lord, I Need You!"

The more often you keep your mind focused on the positive, the easier it becomes—and before long, it just happens without you even thinking about it.

Are you someone who was told as a child you would never amount to anything, or that you were lazy or stupid? Maybe you were told this by a parent, a relative, a friend, or even a teacher. Far too many people have been hurt this way, and they are stuck in a place that is unhealthy because those words have become stuck in their own mind. The very words that hurt you can teach you something even greater. Words are power if we use them wisely. If you believed the negative things that were spoken to you, why can't you believe the positive words about yourself? The truth is that people believe negative things more easily. I think we were all born that way, but we don't have to stay like that.

We have a choice, and since you are reading this, it means you are ready. You have decided you want a different life, and that decision will be all you need to start the healing process. An open mind and heart are the beginning of real, lasting change.

Today is a great day! You are alive! Have you ever thought about the two gifts you open every morning—your eyes?! What about the breath of air you just took—have you ever really thought of that as a precious gift? Truly, just ponder that. Without it, there would be no life. Just like a heartbeat going up and down—it too represents life.

We won't always have mountaintop experiences, and we do need to go down to the valley in order to learn something. It's during hard times that you learn the most about yourself, if you are willing to embrace the lesson life wants to teach you.

Today I want you to start a new mission that will have a wonderful influence in your life. I want you to buy yourself a special journal where you begin a gratitude journey. When you focus on the many blessings and the good things happening around you, it releases more joy into your life. You begin to notice the simpler things in life, and in time you will see them as the big things. I always tell people to start with something that is easy for you to maintain so that you will keep it up every day. Start small and watch how quickly your list begins to grow.

Begin each day by writing down three things you are grateful for. Try to write something different daily, as this makes you become more aware of things that would usually go unnoticed.

For example, in the morning I like to start by giving thanks for the new day I am blessed with. Each day is a new beginning, and we can make it better than yesterday. It's a fresh start! Have you ever been in the shower and your mind is already thinking about work, the kids, or the many things you need to accomplish for the day? You are not really even in the shower. Your mind has checked out, and you are missing so many beautiful blessings right there at that moment. Once you pull your mind back to the present moment, you will begin to appreciate the smells of the shower in the morning, the feelings of warm water washing over your body, and the joy of being cleansed.

When we allow our senses to come alive, we begin to appreciate even more the smells of fresh coffee brewing and that first taste. The mind begins to receive so much more when we open our hearts to receive it. When your day begins in a positive way, reflecting on gratitude, it will only release more joy and give you more to be thankful for. What you sow, you will receive. The more thankful you become, the more you can stay that way throughout the entire day. Before long, you will notice a complete stranger smiling at you from across a room and it will cheer you up instantly, or you may think of someone who held a door for you as you left the store. We are blessed many times throughout a normal day, but our minds are not focused on the present and we miss these wonderful gifts. Once you begin to notice and receive these beautiful acts of kindness, you will be filled with joy and you will want to bring that joy to others. That's how small acts of kindness grow and spread—one at a time. The truth is, once you start to spread some of these seeds in your life, you will start to receive even more joy in your own life too.

In the evening, give thanks for three more things that made your day special. This is the best way to have a good night's rest. A thankful heart is a happy heart, and a mind at peace will rest well. Sweet dreams, my friend.

This is the day the Lord has made. We will rejoice and be glad in it.

—Psalm 118:24

I will praise you, Lord, with all my heart; I will tell of all the marvelous things you have done.

—Psalm 9:1

Forgiveness Is Freedom
Chapter Two

Many people who have been hurt badly by others struggle with forgiveness. I hope that by sharing my own experiences, I can help open your eyes to the larger freedom that forgiveness brings. When I was seventeen years old, I remember taking great offence from some people who claimed to be Christians when they asked me in a doubtful tone if I was one too. Their comments made me feel as if I was being judged for my faith and my path. Why did they feel the need to even ask me this question? That was when I began to build walls around myself so I'd be protected from the judgment of others. Have you yourself had someone in a church or elsewhere make these kinds of harsh judgments against you? I believe that with this behaviour, far too many Christians are hurting unbelievers— as well as their own brothers and sisters in the Church.

Words cause more damage than we realize, and sometimes it takes years to reverse that damage. This happens very often, and it causes people to harden their hearts. This is what happened to me at seventeen, as I believed with all of my heart I was a Christian. I had been raised by both parents, who took all of us kids to church and Sunday school. We said grace and we prayed. I'd been christened as a baby and had given my life to the Lord at a Christian camp at the age of eleven. But the truth is, I didn't have a personal relationship with Jesus. And later as an adult, I came to realize my life didn't reflect the life of a Christian. Why am I sharing this? When we hear another person's story, we come to trust that they can relate to us if we've had the same experiences.

In 2003 my sister Darlene and I had a discussion that didn't end well. In one night, a relationship was destroyed. Again, this shows the power of our words. It only takes one small spark to start a huge forest fire, and the very words we use can destroy as quickly as fire. That evening, there was a fire of words, and as a result, we went four long years without speaking. Sadly, it affected my family as well as the extended family. I was so uncomfortable around my sister that I started to stay away from family functions. As time went on, I realized I was missing out on precious time with everyone else, and the unforgiveness in my life was affecting my mind, body, and spirit. I was becoming ill from it. It was a destructive time in my life. I would keep the offence in my mind by thinking about it often, which only led to a vicious cycle of unhappiness. While I obsessed over our argument, my anger became the words I released into the world. We need to be careful about what we allow our minds to feed upon. I was in a really bad place, and honestly I didn't want to stay there. I didn't like the person I was turning into.

I remember going to my brother, Joe, and sharing how tired all of this was making me. He shared a scripture with me that day: *"So don't worry about tomorrow, for tomorrow will bring its own worries. Today's trouble is enough for today"* (Matthew 6:34). The truth is, we should live our lives one day at a time. Joe told me that when I went to bed that night I should pray and ask God to help me to forgive our sister. With that, he gave me a hug and said a prayer over me.

I will never forget the following morning. When I woke up, I told my husband Ted, "I don't know what Joe did to me last night, but I feel a thousand pounds lighter." Of course, now I understand it was the power of prayer, and the healing had begun the moment I opened my heart. My brother had taught me a very valuable lesson about the power of prayer.

My sister and I had come to a place in our lives where we were able to forgive one another and realize our pride was getting in the way. Pride makes us think our words need to be heard.

I remember asking God one morning while I was driving to work, "What would have happened if I had stayed quiet and not spoken?"

His answer was very simple. *"Nothing."*

From this experience, and from others over the years, I have learned that you have to really ask yourself, "Are the words I am saying going to help the situation or make it worse?" Sometimes the best answer is to stay quiet. If you don't speak, you can't cause an argument. God showed me that when a person says something you may not agree with, as soon as you open your mouth you become 50% responsible for the outcome. Sometimes the wise thing is to agree to disagree. If you learn this very valuable lesson, it will save you a lot of conflict in your relationships too.

You often see this pattern with people who talk a lot: they can't listen to another point of view without becoming defensive. I recognize this in myself, as I was always talking and unable to hear others. Quite often we involve ourselves in other people's business when we don't need to. We may think we are helping them by giving advice or our opinion, but in truth, if we stay quiet we won't get dragged into other people's problems. The most powerful thing we can do is pray for them and let the Spirit show them what He wants them to see.

I give thanks for these hard lessons. I have learned to see myself for who I am, and I've made some wonderful changes that have helped me to stay at peace with everyone around me. The Word teaches us, *"You must all be quick to listen, slow to speak, and slow to get angry"* (James 1:19).

I also learned another valuable lesson from this experience: our children are watching and listening to us. When they see us treating others badly or passing judgement, they begin to believe this is the way they should act too. This is hard for me to share, but I have to remember that there is not a perfect person in this world and we are all broken and lost. As my daughter watched my broken relationship for four years, she wondered why she couldn't see her cousins and play anymore. What kind of message was I teaching her with my behaviour? Of course it affected her. When you watch children play with one another, they may fight over a toy, but they are quick to make up. They don't stay mad, because they haven't learned that yet. What an important lesson my daughter was trying to teach me—don't stay angry for long, as it doesn't help anyone.

Friends, always remember that we too as parents make lots of mistakes while raising our kids. If you want your children to forgive you, then you need to forgive your own parents for some of the mistakes they have made. We can't give away what we don't have inside of us.

I believe now, more than ever, that we can learn from the past. If you saw something that was unhealthy in your life while you were growing up, don't repeat that cycle. Be the "change" in your family and bring up the next generation to learn new ways to love others and treat them well. You can be the change you want to see in the world—but it does start with you first!

Forgiveness is a process that takes time, but when you open the door it allows healing to begin. You will be amazed at the freedom it brings into your life. If God can restore my sister and me to the beautiful place we are today, He can do it for you as well. I am always amazed by how God lines up our ducks in life so that things fall into place in order to benefit us the most. He made sure my relationship with my sister was restored before we headed into the next valley of life. We can't see what's coming tomorrow—and I believe that's a huge blessing, as we are given only what we can handle for today.

Forgiveness is so important and if you only take away one thing from reading this book, I hope you will see how much more lightly you can start living today. People believe they can't forgive someone who has hurt them deeply, because it seems like the other person wins from the injustice they have caused. The truth is, you forgive them to release yourself from the burden.

More often than not, people hurt us with words or actions without even realizing it. Quite often, we ourselves have hurt others unintentionally too. Why do you need to forgive? When you don't let go of the unforgiveness in your heart, it becomes your weight to carry. When you can't let go of bitterness, resentment, jealousy, and anger, they take up space in your spirit. Think of it like a suitcase: the more you hold the pain and hurt, the heavier that suitcase becomes for you to carry. The only way to let it go is to open it up and remove what's weighing it down. Do you want to stay bitter over what someone has done to you in the past and have the possibility of letting it steal your future too? I don't believe anyone wants that. You have a choice, you can change this today and free up space in your spirit for better things like joy, love, and peace to come in. Will it be easy? No, not at all. But will you feel better and lighter in the end? Yes, for sure.

When I was on my mission to find healing, I was given an appointment with someone who did forgiveness coaching with the use of a mirror. I remember the day I arrived, and how I felt like I didn't really have anyone I was angry with or even upset with. I truly couldn't see how this coach was going to help me. But as we began to talk about the past and the different things I had experienced, I saw some of the roots in my own life were deeper than I realized. As we started working through a list of people in my life, I came to see I had scars that I needed some healing from.

I was very surprised at some of the things that came up that day, but this just goes to show that sometimes we are deceived by ourselves, too. Just like the story in the Bible of the prodigal son who left home with his inheritance: he wanted to live his life, his way. When all the money was gone, he returned home asking for his father's forgiveness. He came to understand the truth about his situation. He needed repentance and forgiveness for straying off God's path. On the other hand, his brother struggled with the forgiveness his father gave so easily. He couldn't believe his father would welcome his brother back with a grand celebration, but the father did this because he loved his son. A son who was lost was now found.

We don't talk about the second son much, but I believe many of us are more like him. He thought he was okay—like we do—but in truth he was holding onto resentment and anger. He was jealous that he had stayed home faithfully, yet never received a celebration for all his hard work.

Many of us look at life as an iceberg. We see the problems of others sticking out above the water, but we won't allow ourselves to deal with the root of our own problems below the surface. The truth is, our own problems are just that—ours—until they are dealt with.

Such an event came up for me, and I was shocked because I didn't realize that it was even bothering me. It was deep below the surface of the water. When I was a young girl, my pony Silver had been coughing badly for a few weeks. My daily routine was to run out to his pen to see him after school. One day, he was nowhere to be found. I remember my father telling me he'd sent him away because he was sick.

As the memory came flooding back to me, I burst into tears. I'd never gotten to say goodbye. Now all these years later, this event came up, even though I hadn't realized my own upset emotions towards my father. Why? I believe we bury things that are painful (try to forget them) because we don't want to deal with the pain.

I came home after my appointment and journaled. I began to see that my father probably felt it would be easier on me, which was why he'd chosen to do it this way. He was trying to save me unnecessary pain. Honesty can sometimes be a lot to hear, but in truth, that memory totally set me free. Even though I never realized it, my spirit knew I needed to forgive my dad. I love my dad with all my heart, and I know he did what he thought was best for me.

One woman shared with me that at age four her father thought it was time she grew up and she no longer needed her doll. That day, he threw her doll into the wood stove. As she shared this experience with me, her eyes filled with tears and she said, "It feels like it just happened yesterday. I can still see it happening." This was a woman in her eighties who probably wasn't even aware that she needed to forgive—yet it had been a stronghold in her life for all those years.

As I was writing, I knew the Spirit was asking me to add this part to the book. In truth, I have forgiven the individuals that caused the offence so I didn't intend to share it initially, but by sharing, it may help other women who have struggled in this area. From the time I was around eleven or twelve till the age of sixteen, I was touched inappropriately by three different men. It was something that I never shared with anyone until I met my husband. Why not? Shame and fear. I believe we often blame ourselves for treatment that we didn't deserve in any way.

Ladies, the best way to move past these issues is to open the door for only a moment so you can acknowledge that it happened to you, and forgive the people who hurt you. Once I forgave them, I was able to truly move forward and forget. I now believe the pain I was holding was part of the reason why I was drinking too much: it was a way to forget rather than face the truth head-on. Isn't that true? When we understand ourselves better, it can explain some of the habits or addictions that have become coping mechanisms that we are in denial about.

Sometimes our wounds are much deeper than we realize, and if we don't deal with them they can keep opening up, holding us captive. Do you want to keep going around the same mountains? How do you move forward to forgive someone in your life? I can already hear you asking, "How on earth do I do this?"

If you already know Jesus, it will be much easier because He can give you the ability to do so. Unfortunately, there are far too many Christians who are still struggling in this area, which is truly sad because we are to be a light to others around us. If we can't set an example by doing what God teaches us, then why on earth would anyone else want what we have? In the eyes of nonbelievers, we will seem just as bad as anyone else. Jesus came here to live and set an example for us to follow, so we need to do better. In truth, we are His representatives, so let us work on ourselves before we try to help others. We are all human, but if you are still struggling in this area, ask for help from someone who can guide you along and ask for extra prayers.

If you don't know Jesus yet, don't wait to ask Him for His Help. If you ask, seek, and knock, He will answer you. It's as simple as saying these words: "Jesus, I can't do this alone; will You help me out? I choose to heal from my past pains. I want to forgive anyone and everyone who has ever hurt me in my life, as well as receiving Your healing for every circumstance and every situation I have had to endure."

Who is it you need to forgive? Some of your relationships may never be completely restored to the level of that of my sister and I, but it doesn't mean you can't heal. Sometimes we need to protect our own lives from things that could cause us greater pain down the road, and this is okay. If something is not healthy for you (or someone else) and you recognize it, follow your heart with forgiveness and let it go. I have met people who had pain caused by a family member who hurt them deeply, but they are no longer here. How do you move past this?

Here is something you can do which has wonderful benefits for the process of healing from people and events—in the present as well as in the past. When I use this exercise to help others, I tell them to write down the person's name and the offence they caused. (I would like you to note that I don't hear their stories myself or ask what the person has done to them, as listening to that darkness would hurt my own spirit. I believe many counsellors get burned out because they are exposed to many harsh details which only end up hurting them personally. It can be too much darkness being expelled into the environment we are in, and it becomes unhealthy for everyone. God has taught me that I can help others without hurting myself, and moving them into freedom by doing things a little differently than most would.)

After you have written down the person's name and offence, I encourage you to write a letter to them—don't worry, they won't actually read any of it. I recommend doing this in your own handwriting, as this method is much deeper in your spirit than using a computer. You can describe how they made you feel and how much they hurt you. Always end your letter with the words, "I choose to forgive so that I can be set free."

When I take people through this process, we then go to the firepit where I leave them alone and they read their letter out loud so they can hear themselves say the words.

You can do this on your own. After expressing your feelings and maybe a few tears, you can light your letter on fire. Once you do this, it becomes a prayer to Heaven.

Are you struggling with something in your own life that you can't forgive yourself for? Follow the same guidance, only address the letter to yourself. Choose to forgive yourself and let it set you free. When you take these actions, it is a step of faith that you are connecting with your mind, heart, and hand, that you are willing to release that pain to a higher power. He is the only one who can truly help. God hears every prayer and sees every tear you shed, and He wants to heal you. This is truly just between you and God, who already knows everything about you.

When you are willing to confess, it really does set you free. I believe when we confess our faults to God and to others, no shame, guilt, or fear can ever hold us back again. We are free! I know of people who have actually gone to the gravesite of someone in order to release their forgiveness, which has brought some wonderful healing for them as well.

Friends, we all have pains, and the sooner we deal with them the better off we are in our physical being. Most times, the physical pain we feel in our bodies is truly just a symptom of a deeper cause with a much deeper root. Be set free today and forgive. Say goodbye to your pain, and be encouraged as you keep moving forward with these challenges. It will get easier and you will be thankful that you stuck with it. Keep going!

Accept my prayer as incense offered to you, and my upraised hands as an evening offering.

—Psalm 141:2

Finally, I confessed all my sins to you and stopped trying to hide my guilt. I said to myself, "I will confess my rebellion to the Lord." And you forgave me! My guilt is gone.

—Psalm 32:5

...he will give a crown of beauty for ashes...

—Isaiah 61:3

Loss and Life

Chapter Three

After my sister and I received healing in our relationship, I was so grateful to God. But now there was a valley on the horizon in which our family would have to face a whole new chapter of lessons of pain on love and loss.

In November 2009, my niece Amber (Darlene's daughter) was diagnosed with leukemia. This was a difficult time for a young woman of only nineteen years, as well for her family. She had to undergo many painful procedures and different treatments. One thing that truly amazed me was the joy she was always able to hold, constantly wearing a smile during all she was going through. One thing that stood out in my mind was her request when people wanted to come and visit her—it was that there would be no crying and negative talk in her presence. I believe she understood the value of keeping her environment positive, and this was how she managed to stay so focused and upbeat. She knew the power of the words in her environment could pull her down or build her up.

During this difficult time as I watched my niece fight for her life, I was very abusive with my wine. Truthfully, we all blame our bad habits, choices, or situations we are going through on other people. Whether it's a relationship, health, finances, work, children, or whatever the situation is, we don't like to take responsibility for our own actions. I believe God was trying to speak to me during this time, but I wouldn't listen. I had the earplugs in and didn't want Him to take my wine away.

During those days, I would often ask my husband about faith. I was having a hard time understanding what it really even meant. It was clear that my niece had an amazing faith, and I couldn't get my head around it. How was she able to always show joy in such dark days? I now realize that she was helping me to see through her eyes what faith was.

One evening I was in our hot tub drinking wine and a song was given to me. The words just seemed to come so easily, and I jumped out of the tub so I could quickly write them down before they left my mind. It was a song all about faith. I shared my song with a family friend, and he and his wife were willing to sing and play this song with me on his guitar. I also had the privilege to share it with Amber at a Christmas celebration we had in May 2010 while she was in remission. I believed then that the words were for Amber, but later would come to understand they were for all us—her family. That song and those words were truly a gift from above.

When we lose those we love, it often leaves us asking "Why?" It is such a painful time, and we are never the same afterward. The thing that brings me the most comfort is to know how much Amber loved Jesus and that she had made peace with His decision. I know this to be true, and my life was transformed by watching my niece. I have been changed for eternity.

Who am I to question the way God is moving to touch people? God's ways are not our ways, and His thoughts are not our thoughts, but I do trust each step of the journey He has taken me on. In the end, His plans will show people how much He really does love them. We all have that opportunity of leaving an imprint on another person's soul and guiding them toward a beautiful destination.

The day of Amber's funeral, September 23, 2010, was the day I gave my life completely to God. When I arrived home that night, in the comfort of my bedroom I held my arms in the air and said to God, "I am all Yours now. Use me however You need to so my life will glorify You." Today—and every day—I give thanks for the life of my niece. Without having had her in my life, I may not have gotten to where I am today. Her life touched mine and changed me forever. I believe she had told God that very same thing—that she was willing to let Him use her life to touch another soul. That soul was me.

My life was beginning a whole new transformation, because I was allowing Him to work in all the different areas of my life. His miracle started with me that day at the cottage on May 22, 2011, when I woke up with that painful hangover and He changed me with His touch.

People often ask me, "How did you just quit? Didn't you need to do a twelve-step program or go to some support groups?"

My answer is simple: "No, I just quit."

Many people reply, "How is that possible?" The only answer I can give you is because Jesus touched me that day. I know His hand was on my shoulder, and that He gave me the ability. In the human realm, we aren't able to do these things on our own. It is all *Him*. The word for this is "miracle."

God continued to touch my life when He placed the desire in me to be baptized. Many people couldn't understand why I wanted to be baptized since I'd been christened as a baby. The truth is, when a child is christened, it's the parents making a promise to raise the child up in the faith. It is also an opportunity for the people in the church to promise that they will help guide this family. I wanted to get baptized because I had no memory of my christening, and now, more than ever, I wanted to confirm my faith in an outward expression of what was going on in my heart. I knew God was doing something new in my life.

I was baptized at New Life Community Christian Church in Thornton, Ontario, on April 22, 2012. This was another life-changing day, and I'm so glad I did this in obedience to Him. It was such an empowering moment when I was submerged in the water and came up. I remember feeling a light surrounding me, and I felt like I'd been washed clean from my past. I was a new version of me—I was (Sam) born again.

When we lose those we love, how do we move forward? Who have you lost, and how are you coping? We all know that death is a part of life, but that makes it no easier. But those of us who know where our loved ones are and have the promise of seeing them again can take comfort. There is such great *hope* in that. The thought of seeing my niece again gives me great excitement—that I will be able to thank her for the influence she had on my life. That I will see Heaven one day, and all those I love.

No one knows the day or hour they will depart—only God does. One thing that breaks my heart is when people are sick with a terminal illness and the doctor gives them a timeline. I truly wish they wouldn't do this, as I believe it breaks a person's spirit when they give up hope. I have seen this so many times over the last few years, and it's truly sad. The words the doctors share crush the spirit. Here it is again, friends—the power of *words*.

> *The Lord is close to those who are broken hearted; he rescues those whose spirits are crushed.*
>
> —Psalm 34:18

A friend shared with me that her husband had been very sick with cancer and the doctor gave him only two months.

She asked him to keep his words to himself and let her take her husband home. Her husband knew he was sick, but she wouldn't allow the doctor's words to be heard, as she knew this would break his spirit. She changed his diet and gave him good supplements. After two years, the doctor came by the home to see what she was doing, as he couldn't believe her husband was still living and doing so well. He told her to keep doing what she was doing, and her husband went on to live an additional eight quality years.

Why is it we don't hear these encouraging stores instead of the negative ones? I heard another story of a doctor who got cancer himself. Again, he was told he would be gone within a year. He chose to study the spirit, mind, and body, and see what sense he could make of it. Again, with a change in diet (plant-based) and good supplements, as well as spiritual work, he lived another twenty years. During that time, he continued to experience life and make memories. He was also blessed to see the birth of his son. What did he do with his time? He taught others what he had learned through his life experience, which has helped many people in their fight with cancer. If you are reading this and you are in a battle with some disease where your doctors are giving you no hope, wouldn't you love to hear you have another twenty years?

Another encouraging story I heard was about a woman who was going into surgery. She had cancer, and the family asked if they could stand and pray around her before the surgery. The family stood holding hands and prayed a healing prayer over her, all while the doctor stood in the corner as a witness. There was a screen in the room where everyone could see the mass that they were going to remove. Once the prayer began, the mass began to disappear right in front of the doctor's eyes. He was blown away, and had never witnessed anything like this before. The woman no longer needed the surgery, and she was cancer-free. Miracles happen every day, and we are so blessed when we get to see them for ourselves. I am sure the doctor was changed by that experience, and he will never forget it.

Friends, I once went to a conference for Lyme disease where I had an opportunity to share a few words of hope with the people there. I had been told no one could help me, but I wouldn't let the words of doctors or anyone else stop me from searching for my healing. That was the very hope I shared that day. My words gave people greater *hope*. The words were simple: "If you are sitting today and feel like giving up because you see no hope, with no one wanting to help you, I am here to encourage you. I shouldn't be standing here today—I had even thought of taking too many sleeping pills and stopping the pain. But I chose to keep searching for my own individual answers, because each person has their own DNA and their own healing. There are answers; we just have to keep searching."

Right after I shared these words, a gentleman came up to me and said, "Boy, do I wish my son could have heard you. He took his own life because he had lost *hope*. He couldn't cope any longer because he felt alone."

This was heartbreaking to me. A thirty-year-old man left feeling hopeless because of words that were spoken to him. Shortly after that conversation, I spoke with another individual whose husband had been fighting Lyme disease and had lost his battle. She said she felt his spirit was crushed, and that's what really took him. He had given up and wasted away. He had lost *hope*. Now, these families are enduring life without their loved ones.

When will we learn that *words* are *powerful?* They produce life or death. Another issue has been very heavy on my heart: those people who are suffering from daily pain and are tired of living that way, to the point where they are looking for an assisted death. Friends, I know how hard life can be, especially when you are suffering in terrible pain—but please remember, you are loved so much, and your life has meaning. Don't take the way of the world, but keep searching for alternate answers for treatment and coping. You are so worth it!

So now the question is, how do you cope with your loss? I remember after my father passed, someone said to me that, "Every time we see you smile, we see your father." That brought joy to me that I cannot describe, and it still makes me want to smile all the time. My father is not in my sight any longer, but he is with me when I smile. He lives in my heart and spirit. It is such a comfort to me.

If you lose someone you love, talk about their life. Share what they taught you and how they inspired you. Perhaps you might honour a lost loved one by starting a fund in their memory. Even though they are no longer here, they can still help others bring hope to something that was important to them.

Illness and grief are heavy burdens to live with. If you are able to hold firm to your faith, it will give you more strength to keep going. When you build your strength up in hope, your meter grows even more, giving you more faith. What we see now is not all there is in this world, and we are only here for a short time—a time to learn and a time to grow until we are ready for the next chapter, leading us home to our final destination. Heaven.

The truth is, you have nothing to lose by believing, but everything to lose by not believing. Stop here for a few moments and let those words sink deep into your spirit. Jesus is like the wind: you can't see Him, but you feel Him and you see Him moving in people's lives. Just observe the trees. You can't see the wind, but you see it moving the leaves. That is just like Jesus. There is only one way to Heaven, friends, and it's through a relationship with Jesus. Call out to Him and let Him carry all your burdens. As I end this chapter, it's my prayer that you will see we each have a set amount of time here on earth, and when you have *hope*, it keeps your *spirit strong*. May you be blessed to have even more time and know that God loves you so much. Don't give up your hope, and make each day the best it can be.

"For I know the plans I have for you," says the Lord. "They are plans for good and not for disaster, to give you a future and a hope."

—Jeremiah 29:11

But those who trust in the Lord will find new strength, They will soar high on wings like eagles. They will run and not grow weary. They will walk and not faint.

—Isaiah 40:31

I pray that God, the source of hope, will fill you completely with joy and peace because you trust in him. Then you will overflow with confident hope through the power of the Holy Spirit.

—Romans 15:13

Illness and Lessons

Chapter Four

When Lyme disease came knocking on my door, I had to quit the residential/commercial cleaning business that I had run for eighteen years. It was July 2013, and I was brought down to my knees. I had no energy to do anything, which was extremely hard for me, as I was the kind of person who usually had enough energy for three people. I had nothing left even for myself. I was completely spent and burnt out.

My health had been declining since 2009, when I started to have stomach and bowel issues. I was going from doctor to doctor for all kinds of tests, and was put on many different medications that were only adding to my problems. For the better part of a year and a half, I was being told I had fibromyalgia and chronic fatigue syndrome. At my last appointment in November of 2014, the specialist informed me that they were sorry but they couldn't give me a clear diagnosis.

I remember leaving that appointment feeling absolutely discouraged and hopeless. What was I going to do? I was angry that they had been treating me with all kinds of medications that were causing side effects. As time went on and I began to learn more about gut health, I realized my stomach wall had been completely destroyed.

Many times, we are handed things like business cards, words of wisdom, and even suggestions we should look into.

But often our minds are closed and we are unable to receive what could be an amazing gift. That was me—I had been closed off from receiving.

A memory came flooding back to me in that time of discouragement. I remembered a sister at our church telling me I should look into Lyme disease. She shared that she had seen a lot of articles on it lately. When she heard about my issues, she wondered if this could be the very thing I was struggling with. I remember her giving me newspaper articles that I read, but I didn't make the connection until much later. I am so happy that she came to me to share her thoughts—otherwise I might still be in bed suffering.

Every day, people living on earth serve as messengers for the divine power above, but we don't truly listen. It wasn't long after this experience when I began to pray hard that God would direct my feet on His path so that I could get answers for my failing health. One of my sisters (Christine) gave me the name of a naturopath doctor in Barrie, and I set up an appointment with him right away. Again, another messenger that led me to the hope I needed—the hope of better days coming. I remember how my belief meter began to rise, hoping that all my searching would lead me back to a life that I would one day again enjoy. I remember telling my husband Ted that I would sooner have a quality of life than quantity—to enjoy whatever time God was going to bless me with, and be filled with His joy.

I will always be grateful to Dr. Yarish, who was the person who began my journey of getting my gut healthy. He began working with me through diet and building my immune system with vitamin treatments through IV, "So my body could do its job to fight for me," as he always said. He opened my eyes to see my health in a new light, which only made me want to research even more for myself. Dr. Yarish will never truly realize what he gave me through his gifts. His life has touched mine, and he gave me hope for my health journey.

Right before Christmas 2014, my blood work came back from IGeneX in California, and I learned that I indeed had Lyme disease. To be honest, I was so thankful to learn this, because at least now I knew what I was fighting. I remember thinking many times before this that I was going to die of some unknown disease (my mind was in a very negative state). I even remember wishing it was cancer. You may think it sounds very harsh, but I knew that in Canada there would be no financial or medical help for Lyme disease. Ted and I knew we were really on our own. I was terrified of what this would do to us financially as well as to our relationship. When someone is sick, that is more than enough to worry about without adding the burden of finding financial resources.

Later on, though, this whole experience became the one I am most grateful for. "How?" you might ask. The truth is, it made me see our resources with a new perspective. You can have all the money in the world, but if you haven't got your health, you have nothing. I remember telling Ted I didn't care what it cost us or what we had to do in order for me to become well. That was my mission. I looked at it as an investment so that I could work on my true mission in life.

I believe there are many people who are given a remission in their health so they can remember what the true mission is—to bring more hope to more people who are suffering. If you are reading this today and you have had some setbacks in your health, don't let your financial resources force you to settle for the prescription you can receive for free from a doctor due to your health benefits. I say this because I was that very person—I wouldn't spend our resources to get healthy, but rather preferred to go the route that was covered by healthcare or our insurance company. Don't forget—you are worth the investment, and your life is your greatest asset! Let your resources work in your favour, and do whatever it takes to find your healing answers.

Please hear me when I say this: you know your body better than anyone else. We are all created differently, and we all have different DNA. What works for one person may not work for another, but we will all receive answers if we never give up! Your body is your own responsibility. It's up to you to understand exactly what you're putting into it, and what it is doing to your whole being. Everything from medications, food, drinks, and supplements to what you will allow yourself to listen to and allow yourself to see is your responsibility. (I will go deeper into how food affects not only our bodies, but also our minds and our spirits in another chapter.) You only get one body here on earth, and if you want to enjoy the journey, you can start by caring deeply for the temple you live in. The flesh can easily take us off course, but the spirit wants to lead each one of us on a path that will give us true life and happiness.

Are you sitting here at this moment knowing you need to change a few things to create a healthier life? Are you willing and ready to make a commitment to yourself? If you write down today's date, you will look back on it later as a great day! The first step to healing is making a decision and not having an excuse to stop you from receiving that gift.

Have you been just settling with the words that others have given you like it is your final diagnosis without investing your time, resources, and energy to do your own searching? Be encouraged, friends: if you are suffering from disease, anxiety, depression, financial stress, addiction, or relationship strains, you will have power when you decide to take care of yourself. When you are healthy, you are better able to cope with the everyday things that are going on in your life with a peaceful mindset.

I want to encourage you to keep visuals around your home. If you want to see your health get better, surround yourself with images and objects that keep your mind focused on the positive things you hope to see happen. If you are struggling with a relationship, put words and pictures around that encourage you to keep working at it. If your finances are a mess, keep your focus on seeing that debt coming down penny by penny. Maybe you want to lose some weight—keep pictures of healthy food in your vision with exercise equipment. If you are battling a disease, put images of places you want to go, healthy food, and a picture of yourself before you fell ill. When we see things visually, it keeps our minds in the right place. What we see every day gives us hope, and if we believe all things are possible, it makes it possible.

Something I love using is a vision board. When I was still healing, I had these all over the house, and they kept me inspired that better days were coming. I still do this today. Start your vision board by cutting out pictures from magazines, and fill the page with words that inspire you. The words you say and see will keep your vision first in your mind, which helps to keep you in a positive place so God can work in you. Here are a few words and phrases you could include on your vision board to help build more hope.

Love—Healing—Power—Faith
Hope—Family—Friends—Eyes on Jesus
Peace—Be Still—Balance—Listen
Joy—Life—Confidence
Patience—Trust—Believe
Hugs—Care—Never Give Up

What type of pictures could you use? Whatever inspires you. Maybe for you, it's:

the great outdoors—a campfire—a hike
a bike ride—a sunset—a sunrise
a run—a lake—a dream vacation
a fur baby—mountain top—family/friends
holding hands—playing with children

Friends, material things are just that: material. When we start using our minds to focus our joy on the simpler things, like experiences, we learn of a whole other joy: *one that is born inside of our spirits.* Have fun with this mission, and let it fill you with a much deeper excitement. As people say, seeing is believing. The truth is, in God's eyes it's the exact opposite. Believing is seeing. Some things you may never see unless you believe them first. When you make your vision board, it is because you believe God is working. That is where the power lives in Jesus.

Faith shows the reality of what we hope for; it is the evidence of things we cannot see.

—Hebrew 11:1

Look straight ahead, and fix your eyes on what lies before you.

—Proverbs 4:25

Let all that I am wait quietly before God, for my hope is in him.

—Psalm 62:5

And the Lord answered me and said, Write the vision and engrave it so plainly upon tablets that everyone who passes may [be able to] read [it easily and quickly] as he hastens by.

—Habakkuk 2:2 (AMPC)

Side Trip

Chapter Five

It was January 2015, and I wasn't sure if I should go to the USA to see what kinds of more aggressive treatment were available for my condition. Many people around me told me I should go, and at that time my cognitive functioning was in rough shape. Lyme disease had many wild effects on me, and not only on my mind and body—it really threw me off in the deepest part of my soul. I was in a bad place. I had a very negative attitude and I didn't really believe I could become well again. Now I understand why I was in this dark place. The truth is, I wouldn't allow myself to believe for something better.

We made the trip to the States and it took everything out of me. At that time, I was spending up to eighteen hours a day in bed, and I had no idea how I'd be able to make the big drive to Plattsburgh, New York. My husband and my oldest sister Sylvia made the journey with me. We had to limit the driving time, as I couldn't sit for long without experiencing extreme bodily discomfort. The exhaustion kept me longing to lie down in my bed—I just wanted to be at home in my safe place. I truly didn't like the person I was on this trip, as my pain was taking over my mouth. At times it felt like it wasn't even me speaking. I was losing the person I once was.

I remember praying a lot, asking for the ability to stay quiet and make the best of this trip while my pain was unbearable. I had the most debilitating head pain I could ever describe. It felt like someone was blowing up a balloon in my head and that it was about to pop. My body pain was everywhere, especially in my legs. My mind couldn't find words, and my thoughts weren't coming out the way I intended them to. I was truly a mess.

We had our doctor's visit, but there were many mishaps along the way. I began to believe that I had made a mistake coming all this way. Something inside of me was telling me I'd gone off course, and I began to lose my peace. We ended up coming home with eight weeks' worth of treatment, but after only six weeks of being extremely sick, I gave this treatment up. It took everything good that remained in me and left me completely depleted. My immune system was destroyed. I will never truly know for sure, but I believe everything happens for a reason. Perhaps that treatment was like a kick start, but in the end, I knew I had to do something differently. My body was telling me I couldn't continue this treatment.

During this time, I felt like I was dying from the inside out. That's the only way I can describe the feeling. I had a conversation with Ted and told him, "I need to find a way to do this so I can enjoy the journey while I am making my way down this road of pain." I found during these times I prayed more than ever, and I began to write songs to help me keep control of my anxiety and depression, and make sure my mind was in a good place.

Without God and my faith, I don't believe I could have made it through. Remember how I had considered taking too many pills and going to sleep for good? This shows you the state my mind was in. As time went on, I began to realize these thoughts were coming from the pain medication the doctors had me on. After I made this connection (from watching a commercial and doing some research), I decided to stop taking the pills, and those suicidal thoughts left me. It makes me wonder how many people out there are struggling with the very thing I did. What if your depression is only your medication speaking? Friends, please do your own research and listen to your own body.

While I was struggling with my own illness, my dad's health had started to decline. I was nowhere ready to face that on top of everything else. My dad was a person I always felt very close to, and I could talk to him about anything. On November 24, 2015, my father went home to his eternal home in Heaven. My life would be completely different. I'd always known that I would miss my dad, but I'd never known heartache like that before. He was the head of our family, and an amazing man who taught me so very much. He was very quiet, but he shared so much wisdom. He taught me the most by just living his life. He set an example every day, and he often shared advice and then let us make our own choices.

That's how I believe we all learn: by making mistakes and then—hopefully—being changed by them. Some mistakes are painful, but if they help us become better people, it makes the lesson even more valuable.

I remember one day when I was upset about something and dropped by the house to talk to Dad. He said these words to me: "Sam, how about you go home and when you have calmed down, come back and we will talk about it." That day I felt like a dog with my tail between my legs and head hung down low. When I got home, I stood at my kitchen window and looked down at my parents' home on the corner of the farm property. At that moment, I was able to understand what he was teaching me: that I shouldn't speak when I'm upset or I may say something I'll regret later. Such wisdom again about the power of our words.

I miss my dad more than words can ever say, but I know that he is always with me. Fortunately, before he passed away,

I had been praying that I could have some quality alone time with my dad, and God answered that prayer. At Christmas the year before he passed, I went to him and asked if I could write his memoirs. I thought it would be wonderful to have some stories from his childhood saved for his descendants. This time was one of my most treasured memories with my dad. We sat for hours over coffee as I took down notes and listened to his stories. One day in the kitchen of our farmhouse, he broke down in tears. I had never seen my father cry before, and he wanted to share some words with me that brought more understanding into my own life. He shared these words: "I hope all of my kids know how much I truly love you and that I am proud of each one of you." He said, "Your mom and I did the very best we could with what we had."

After his words were out, I had to respond. I said, "Dad, I believe you did a great job, and we all know you love us." Looking back now, I believe my father's words were healing for him to say, as they were for me to hear. There are no perfect families or people, because we are all human. The wisdom my father shared with me was that we are all doing the very best we can.

Grief is terrible, and there is no right or wrong way to grieve. Everyone does it differently, and there is no timeline. Time doesn't heal all wounds, but we learn to live with our grief, and I do believe my dad would want all of us to go on living and enjoying our lives. That's just the way he was. His mind was always on others, not himself. Even in the last moments of his life, he was asking his granddaughters how their jobs were and about their boyfriends. His focus was still on everyone else.

There is a great deal of wisdom to learn from that. If we keep our focus off ourselves and take an interest in others, it keeps us in a place of humility. Many times, our focus on our own lives or problems makes us self-absorbed. One of the best ways to combat this is to do something for someone else. When we do so, it keeps our minds off ourselves so that we can help others, which releases even greater joy in our own lives. I am truly thankful that God gave me such a loving earthly father. Not everyone has had that blessing in their life.

Some of you may not even know who your father was, or perhaps you lost your father at a young age. Maybe your dad was abusive or had an addiction that turned him into a violent man. For some of you, it may be that your dad just never connected on a level that you longed for. Maybe you wish he could have spent more time with you to make some beautiful memories. Or maybe your father just walked away from your family, leaving you to grow up without a dad and leaving a small hole in your heart.

I know many who have found the comfort that they need from their Heavenly Father, and if you don't know Him, my prayer is that you too will find this comfort. We all have a story of where we have come from, and while no two stories are the same, we do have hope of healing some of those old wounds if we will allow it to happen.

What is your story? How do you cope with the things that are bothering you right now? Do you talk about them with someone you trust? Are you keeping the pain alive by ruminating on the offence? Are you struggling with a decision you need to make regarding a relationship, finances, health, or some other big issue in your life?

When I was a little girl of only ten years, I began to journal. All these years later, I still journal, and I believe it has been a true blessing in my life. As time has gone on, I have learned a great deal about myself from the pages that I read about my past—I have truly grown and changed over the years. I believe journaling helped me to cope with my feelings, and though I didn't realize it until a few years ago, I was actually writing prayers. It's pretty cool looking back to see how far I have come from something that was bothering me—how I worked through my own heartache or pain on the pages between the lines.

I want to encourage you to start to write something every day: write about something that is bothering you, and allow yourself to feel. It's important to know what you are feeling. Identify it. Is it fear, anger, sadness, hopelessness, resentment, happiness, excitement, or something else? Today, more than ever, many people are put on medications that don't allow them to feel their own emotions. Yes, there are times people need medicine, but could we be helping ourselves by using this simple technique?

The connection from the mind, heart, and hand has an amazing power to release those emotions. This allows you to let go of the things that have a grip on you. Once you start to do this, after a while you will be able to look back on a timeline that shows what you have come through. I believe too many people are holding things in their lives that are holding them back and are no longer serving them. Truthfully, it is actually hindering their walk. I've had people express their fear that someone may read what they have written in their journals when they are gone. My response to that—would that be so bad? Perhaps it would help the next generation to understand what you were going through, and help them better understand themselves. If this fear is stopping you from journaling, then you may need it even more. That fear is keeping you stuck, and once you allow yourself this gift, you will feel your spirit soar.

This is your life, and you get to decide when you are ready to move forward. Sometimes we have to pick up the pieces we are left with, even if we aren't totally happy with how things have turned out in our lives. When that time comes and you are ready to take those pieces and build something different and new, you can and you will.

The only true way to keep moving forward is one step at a time. One day at a time. When you renew your mind daily, it creates an environment that will allow you to look forward to the good things that God wants you to receive. Will you allow the good stuff to come in? If you are ready now, then say these words out loud and take action by holding your hands up, showing you believe in the promise of faith: "I am ready and willing to receive all the good things you want me to have, and I give you thanks for them. Amen."

Every good and perfect gift is from above, coming down from the Father of the heavenly lights, who does not change like shifting shadows.

—James 1:17 (NIV)

Don't copy the behavior and customs of this world, but let God transform you into a new person by changing the way you think. Then you will learn to know God's will for you, which is good and pleasing and perfect.

—Romans 12:2

Ways of Healing

Chapter Six

As we begin this chapter, I want to share a few things my daughter Ashley taught me about the importance of listening. Yes, listening again. I believe she was being used as a messenger to share some wisdom with me.

"Mom, do you know people can appear to be listening without actually hearing anything?" she asked.

Because we get so distracted with our life, we often stop listening. Sometimes our children have real wisdom to share, but we aren't willing to learn. I thank Ashley for so many valuable things she has taught me. The truth is, as long as we have a willing heart to learn, we will. No matter our age, we should learn something new every day. It has taken me a long time to learn how to *be still* so I can hear with my *spiritual ears,* but I'm so thankful that God has sent other people to teach me these things.

Healing comes in many different forms. While it can happen all at once, more often it takes time. Through my journey, I could actually feel when I was receiving some healing, and it is absolutely remarkable when it comes. Often, thinking about it can bring me to tears as I contemplate how amazing God is. He uses different methods for different people, and He does want to help you, so open your heart and allow Him to start the process.

I will divide this chapter into sections to share my experience and give you hope that you too can receive the same healing.

Prayer

The first and most important thing you need in your life is prayer. If you humble yourself, admit and repent of your sins, and come to the throne to ask for help, He is ready to step in.

When my journey began, I had a really bad attitude. I was stuck in my illness. Honestly, I was having a pity party for myself. I felt alone and had no real hope of getting better, because I was listening to the wrong voice. The voice of darkness comes to deceive people and make them feel hopeless by filling their minds with lies.

We knew Canada didn't offer treatment for Lyme disease because it is not a recognized disease here (as of March 2020). There is still a lot of medical confusion as to the standard for testing, treatment, and education in Canada. It's my prayer that things are going to change for those who are suffering. The funny thing about Lyme disease is that even though they don't recognize it, if you have a tick on your body, they will treat you with a course of antibiotics. If you catch this disease in the first thirty days, it can be treated. It is a complicated disease, but in time we are hopeful the government will recognize it and help with treatment.

We knew it was going to be a real battle to get my health back on track. I will always be grateful to the church family at the Ivy Presbyterian Church in my hometown. One Sunday, my sister Kathy asked if a few church members could come down and pray with me. I was truly grateful for this gesture, as I wasn't in a good place.

The pastor, his wife, my brother, my sister-in-law, and my sister came to our home and prayed for me. When they arrived, I was a bit uneasy as I hadn't experienced anything like this before. At first, I thought it was strange to be anointed with oil and have prayers of healing spoken over me, but I could tell something was happening to me at that moment. I knew I was receiving healing.

If I'd been listening to the wrong voice, I wouldn't have accepted this gift of prayer.

After that experience, I had a much better attitude toward my illness and felt more hopeful than ever before. I was also filled with more peace. I knew God would work on my behalf, guiding my steps from that day forward.

Maybe you're feeling the very same way today—feeling stuck in your situation and not knowing how to move forward. If so, I encourage you to ask for help. The truth is, asking for help isn't a sign of weakness but rather a sign of strength.

If people would like to pray with you or for you, allow this precious gift. Prayer is a privilege that connects us to the power of the one true Healer. I often say that prayer is like a lamp. If the lamp isn't plugged into the power source, you can't receive the light. We are the same way: if we won't plug into God's light, then we can't receive His power to change the difficult situations we're going through.

God's word is a lamp to our feet and a light for our path, and He will show us the way forward if we keep asking. In His word, He says,

> *And so I tell you, keep on asking, and you will receive what you ask for. Keep on seeking, and you will find. Keep on knocking, and the door will be opened to you. For everyone*

> *who asks, receives. Everyone who seeks, finds. And to every-*
> *one who knocks, the door will be opened.*
>
> —Luke 11:9–10

The real fruit comes from what God sees you doing. When you pray, ask God to send you to the right doctors, to use medicine to heal you, and to strengthen your faith for your journey. Many of you already know of the power of prayer, but if you didn't grow up understanding the reason people pray, I hope you will feel encouraged and be willing to bring your needs before God. I have faith that if you try, you will be amazed at the hope it brings you.

Water

Number two on my list is water. Water is life in the physical world, just as it is in the spiritual world. Most people don't realize that we are mainly made up of water, so drinking water is critical to many aspects of the body.

Did you know that you should be drinking half of your body weight in ounces every day? For example, if you weigh 150 lbs, you should be drinking at least seventy-five ounces per day. How are you doing in this area?

Friends, water does the body so much good. It is life. It keeps us hydrated and helps in other ways, such as by flushing toxins out of the body. We eliminate toxins through our bladder, bowels, and sweat. If we are not drinking enough water, we run into problems and the body cannot function the way it was intended to. Those toxins begin to build up in the body. If we are not detoxing our body every day properly, we will start to experience more body pain. Water also keeps our muscles, cells, and joints properly lubricated so they move more freely.

What about the spiritual water we all need? How do you quench your thirst when it comes to spiritual matters? We can all drink freely from the Bible, and hear me when I say this: the more you draw from this well, the more you will desire to drink it. It will become more thirst-quenching than physical water. To begin drinking your spiritual water, start with one scripture a day and just bathe in it. Soak in it and let it become real in your life.

For those who struggle drinking physical water, here are a few ideas to help you. Set the timer on your phone to remind you it's time to drink. If you don't really like to drink water, try boiling up some flavoured teas and chilling them. Another idea is to simply add some lemon, limes, cucumber, fresh mint, or even basil to your water for some great flavour. Many people can't drink water because it's too cold; try drinking it at room temperature. But do your very best to start drinking more each day. You will start to see many benefits from something so simple.

Food

The third thing we need to talk about is food. These days, our world is so out of balance in this area. We have all gone the way of convenience and speed, but at the cost of something much greater—our health.

Today we see more disease and mental health issues than ever before. As the old saying goes, "You are what you eat." The more I learn about food and gut health, the more grateful I am for this knowledge. When we are learning, it offers us hope that we can change the things that need changing if we are to be brought to a much better place. Knowledge is power if we don't turn a blind eye to it.

In a world where so many chemicals are being added to our food—pesticides and sprays, environmental toxins, and preservatives—and we're eating more fast food and processed food than ever, is it any wonder we are getting sicker every year? Our bodies are not designed to withstand this abuse. Our society is also addicted to sugar, which is a huge problem, creating a vicious cycle of illness and body pain.

I am amazed at how often people I speak with will tell me they don't eat much sugar at all. When I hear this, I see they don't have much knowledge on the subject, as I didn't when I first fell ill. I was told to drop all the sugar from my diet in order to repair my gut wall. I had candidiasis, which many people have without being aware of it. This is a condition in which the lining of the stomach is leaking from the gut into the body due to a fungal infection caused by a type of yeast called Candida. There are many people (including me at the beginning of this process) who don't understand that Candida overgrowth can start from taking antibiotics, a diet high in sugar and refined carbs, high alcohol intake, a weakened immune system, taking oral contraceptives, diabetes, and high-stress levels. When Candida begins to be overproduced, it can lead to various health problems. Major signs include bloating in the stomach, problems with digestion, and bowel issues. To start the healing process, I had to cut out all sugar and stick to vegetables in order to repair my stomach wall.

Going through this process for six weeks really opened my eyes. When I began to read food labels, I realized that everything has sugar in it. The label lists the ingredients in order of prevalence. For example, if you see tomatoes and then sugar, you know that tomatoes are the primary ingredient and that sugar is the second-largest ingredient. The sugar we consume is not just that added teaspoon in your coffee; it is also in potatoes, pasta, bread, crackers, etc. These foods turn to sugar in the body. So let me ask you: how much sugar are you really consuming?

Friends, I hope this helps open your eyes so you will begin to take an interest in what you are allowing into your body. When we are giving the body sugar, it keeps us sick. Sugar feeds many diseases, as I learned. It was feeding my Lyme disease, and it is also a huge factor for people fighting cancer. It's a vicious cycle that keeps people sick and in terrible pain. Do you suffer from more aches and pains than you used to? Sugar holds inflammation in the body, so you can help stop the aches and pains you are feeling by simply cutting out sugar.

Would it be worth it to give up sugar with the reward of less body pain? They say sugar is worse than cocaine addiction. How does that make you feel? Would you allow cocaine, another white powdery substance, into your body? If you need help staying away from sugar, just remember what it is doing to your body, and remember it is the same colour as cocaine.

The good seeds we sow in our own lives will reap a wonderful harvest if we just make an investment with our time, resources, and commitment. What about your daily spiritual bread? Are you getting something wholesome to feed your soul? My sister Kathy gave me a daily devotional called *Our Daily Bread*. It tells a brief story about life experience and then links it to the Bible in a way you can understand. After each devotional, there is a scripture to look up, and I can tell you once I started to open my Bible daily and dig into Scripture, it became the bread that fed my soul. It gave me the nourishment that only the Bible can give. It really is the only self-help book you need. It teaches you truth, wisdom, and discernment, which you can apply to your life.

If you don't own a Bible, I encourage you to reach out to someone and ask them for advice on what kind of Bible to buy. I felt very blessed, as I was given a Bible that is easy to understand and has footnotes to help explain the scriptures so I am able to digest what I am reading. Since getting this translation, the Bible became more real to me because I could relate it more easily to my life. Start simply by reading one scripture a day, and see where it takes you. Your hunger will grow naturally, and it will become a portion of food that truly satisfies.

Music

We all know that music can calm us down with soft relaxing sounds or pump us up if we want to do a workout or need extra energy. But music is so much more than just nice sounds. It contains power.

I once received a message from my husband's cousin Reid, who knew I loved music. He asked me if I would be interested in listening to some healing music that he had. He really felt it could help me in my recovery. I told him I was open to trying anything if it might help me to heal. I got excited, and couldn't wait to receive this music so I could start to listen to it right away.

The day it arrived, I was shocked to see it included seven CDs and a book called *Wholetones: The Sound of Healing* by Michael S. Tyrrell, sharing the story of how he had been able to create this music. Michael's music works at the cellular level through different frequencies which are truly a gift from God, and I could feel it. I began to listen right away, playing the CDs a lot in the car, as well as in our home and cottage. I did this for a couple of months. I really enjoyed the music and it truly did relax me.

One day I had someone mention to me I should try this healing group that was sharing a type of meditation with music. I didn't jump at the offer because I always like to run everything past Jesus first to make sure it's the path He wants me to take. As I was praying to Him, I asked Him about trying the meditation class.

His answer was very simple: "No, you already have everything you need. Music is all you need."

When I heard His quiet soft voice in my heart, I knew He was speaking about the Wholetones music. I grew more excited as He told me I needed to be intentional with Him and this music. I was supposed to be going away with Ted that weekend to meet some friends, but I felt simply exhausted. I knew I was to stay back and soak in the presence of the Lord and be still with this music.

As I look back at the way things happened, it makes me think of the story of Martha and Mary. Mary chose to sit at Jesus's feet and listen attentively to His words. Instead of trying to busy herself like Martha, she chose to sit quietly and experience something far greater than the physical food—she chose to nourish her heart with His spiritual food. This music was the spiritual food I needed. The week leading up to that Saturday, I re-read the entire book that had come with the CDs. I was dedicating my day to the Lord, and I knew something amazing was going to happen—but I had no idea just how awesome it would be!

I know the decision to stay home was planned by God, and I will never forget that amazing day as long as I live. August 13, 2016, I got up in the morning and prepared my heart and mind to just *be still*. I started with the first CD called "Open Door" to prepare my heart to receive. I started by sitting down on the floor and taking a few deep breaths. I listened to all seven CDs—22:22 minutes each. After each one I would write down what I had experienced. At one point, I felt my body begin to tingle. Every CD I listened to affected me differently, but there were three frequencies that were speaking to my body in a wonderful way.

The next one, called "Transformation," was at 528 HZ—
the frequency for DNA. At this point, something happened to
me. My entire body was tingling. I had already lain down on my
back as I was tired of sitting. As I lay there alone in the house absorbing the music, my body felt paralyzed from the chest down.
I couldn't feel anything, and it was almost hard to breathe.
My body was very heavy. I just lay there, wondering what was
happening to me. I knew this was going to be the beginning of
something even better than I could have ever imagined.

That day, I just kept listening to the music over and over,
and then I would journal some more. I was stirred to listen
to the music once again while reading through the book, it
seemed like even more things were being revealed to me. I had
been digging into the scripture that day along with the music
and things seemed to come alive—meanings I hadn't understood before, but which were now beginning to make sense.
These verses became very real to me:

> *And so I tell you, keep on asking, and you will receive what
> you ask for. Keep on seeking, and you will find. Keep on
> knocking, and the door will be opened to you. For everyone
> who asks, receives. Everyone who seeks, finds. And to every-
> one who knocks, the door will be opened.*

—Luke 11:9–10

While this scripture was speaking to me, memories came
flooding back to me of when Ted and I had climbed a fire tower in a town not far from our cottage. I remember that day my
legs wouldn't bend well from Lyme disease so I couldn't do
the whole climb, but I was able to go halfway up and Ted went
to the very top. We had both taken pictures, and it gave me a
whole new perspective on how the view from the same place

can look very different due to the elevation of where the viewer is standing. Our view was the same, but different.

I knew that revelation would play a part in something down the road to help me understand something even more clearly. When we had come down from the tower, we had a conversation with the woman who worked in the store. She had shared with us that some city folks had come to see the moose in Algonquin Park, and were rather disappointed that they had not seen anything on their journey. They thought it was going to be a place where they could pull in and see the moose without searching. They never realized they would be driving through the park with the hopes of seeing some moose. This story made me think of us as humans—so often, we want things to happen without any work involved. But "faith" is an action word that requires us to do something. A scripture that speaks to me, *"Ask me and I will tell you remarkable secrets you do not know about things to come"* (Jeremiah 33:3).

The day that I was lying there on the floor with the music, another Bible verse came to my mind.

For she thought to herself, "If I can just touch his robe, I will be healed." Immediately the bleeding stopped, and she could feel in her body that she had been healed of her terrible condition.

Jesus realized at once that healing power had gone out from him, so he turned around in the crowd and asked, "Who touched my robe?"

His disciples said to him, "Look at this crowd pressing around you. How can you ask, 'Who touched me?'"

But he kept on looking around to see who had done it. Then the frightened woman, trembling at the realization of what had happened to her, came and fell to her knees in front of him and told him what she had done. And he said to her,

> *"Daughter, your faith has made you well. Go in peace. Your suffering is over."*
>
> —Luke 5:28–34

I began to realize what was happening to me. It was time to let go of the old Sam. It was a process I refer to as "grieving the loss of the woman I once was." I knew if I didn't say goodbye to the old Sam, I wouldn't be free to move into the new Sam. I was being healed, but I had to allow it. The old Sam was the one filled with loads of energy, and now it was time to let her go. I knew my energy might not ever be the same, and I had been allowing that thought to stop the healing from coming in. The whole message was this: concentrate on the present and enjoy the gift of the present day right now where you are.

That was the day true healing began in my spirit, and I knew it was going to lead me into further healing of my body. *Thank you, Father—I live amazed by you!* After the whole experience with the healing music, I wanted to share what had happened with my mom and oldest sister. If I had gone with Ted, we would have been visiting with them, but I wanted them to *see* what God had done after I'd been obedient by staying home.

The following day I called my mom and sister to share what I had gone through. When I began to explain the whole experience to them, the feeling of being paralyzed from the chest down, my sister gasped, "Do you remember about a month ago when I called you to share what my friend wanted me to tell you?"

I remembered her calling, but asked her to refresh my mind.

"She wanted me to tell you that she has been praying for you, and for some reason, she felt she needed me to tell you that something heavy was going to lift off your chest, and it would be coming soon!" she replied.

I was blown away. I did remember the conversation, but I had never really let it sink down into my soul. I had never met this woman, but I knew she was a Christian and was very attuned to listening. It was a confirmation that the feeling I'd had in my living room was not my own imagination, but was truly a gift from God.

Our cousin Reid was also used as a messenger from God. He is another person for whom I will always be eternally grateful, and I look forward to giving him a big squeeze when I arrive in Heaven. Through his obedience in sending me this music, I am able to share this with you. The Word says, *"Let us find a good musician to play the harp whenever the tormenting spirit troubles you. He will play soothing music, and you will soon be well again"* (1 Samuel 16:16).

Friends, this music is a gift from above. It has helped people who suffer from health ailments fight anxiety and depression, and it has even helped animals. Take some time to learn what you can, and remember, those with an open mind and heart are the ones who can receive freely. (For more, see the contact information at the back of the book.)

Touch

The power of touch is another important avenue toward healing, and many people are working on earth who have been given beautiful gifts in this area. I was handed a business card by my sister Christine (another messenger from God), who had found a woman who offered different services in therapy. Again, I give thanks that when people have shared answers to my prayers with me, I have followed through by doing my part as directed by Jesus.

I made the call and set up an appointment to meet this beautiful soul, Irena. We have grown to be very close friends over these past years, and I believe she is my angel on earth. When I had so much body pain and depletion of strength, she was able to work with me and lead me out of pain. I will always be grateful to her, and I know God is using this beautiful person every day to help others.

When I first met Irena, I knew we had a connection, and the rest was history. As she worked with me, she was taking many different courses, and she has developed her own personal treatment involving many different therapies. She does it all: reflexology, head massage and other types of massage, pressure points, and one that was a huge asset for me, lymphatic drainage. There is so much that people don't understand about their immune system and how the lymphatic system works directly with it. Irena knew my immune system was very weak, and I needed as much help as I could get. Even today I can tell when my body is beginning to slow down, and it's a sign my lymphatic system is needing some work. I call it "my regular tune-up" to keep my body working at its best so I can stay strong and do the things I need to do.

Always be listening to the ideas of others and be open-minded, as it could be your answered prayer they are handing you.

Creativity and Art

As time went on, Irena kept encouraging me to take an art class with her, but it was almost a year before I would commit to this adventure. During this time in my life, I was locking myself away from everyone. But after my experience with Michael's music, I began to believe God wanted me to do this art class with her. I believed He was yet to reveal something new to me.

It was an art class where you use a hot iron and press melted crayons onto card paper. I did three pictures that evening, and before I had even decided to go, I had already journaled the colours I would use in my picture.

This artwork is actually quite fascinating. You melt the crayon on a hot iron and set the iron on the paper any way you wish and lift. You then clean off your iron and continue on with another colour. As I kept doing this, I saw what looked to be a mess of colours. In the first two pictures, I didn't really see much and I wasn't satisfied—it felt like something was missing. Still, I kept at the second picture, looking, searching for something.

With the third picture, I was so excited because it seemed to capture the colours in the way I wanted to express myself. It felt like there was a message. It made me think of a vision I'd had one time in the dentist's chair, and a vision was exactly what I was hoping for. As I stared into this picture, I knew something else was there, but I couldn't quite see it.

One of the ladies who was taking the class leaned over to me and said, "That one represents you well." I wasn't sure why she would say that to me, as I had just met her for the first time that evening. She kept looking into the picture and then said to me, "Don't you see it?"

"See what?"

"Do you see the cross?"

I was blown away. When I first looked at this picture, I couldn't see anything but colours. But it hit me instantly at that moment—now I could see what she was looking at! There was a beautiful cross staring right back at me.

How many times in our lives do we stare at something and totally miss the message it holds for us? I knew that evening the message from God was that you really have to seek to find what you are looking for—it won't just happen. You have to keep asking and knocking.

I knew God was going to have an amazing story to go along with this quest. I thought, *How could this woman know this picture represents me well?* I began to wonder if she had read my first book *The Story of My Life: My Cup of Poison*. I never did find out if that was the case, but I knew her comment meant something. My mind went back to the fire tower and the man who was searching for the moose. I knew this all was making sense.

The following day at my treatment with Irena, she asked me, "Did you find what you were looking for?" I was surprised by the question. "Last night you looked like you were looking for something and you had gone very deep within. You just looked like you were searching for something," she continued.

I smiled and said, "Yes I was, and I know one day it will all make sense to me."

Sometimes people will give us ideas to help us, but we just can't hear them. I believe God sends people into our lives as His messengers, but we just can't see it. I was so glad I finally listened, as I know He was trying to use Irena as my messenger. I would also like to thank Patty, our art teacher. God has also used Patty and this amazing artwork to help me see things more clearly. If you ever have the opportunity to try this artwork, go for it.

I challenge all of you to move out of your comfort zone and try something that is creative. We all have it in us—we just need to release it and allow more joy into our lives. If we would do more of the things we used to do as children, we would enjoy our lives even more. Life is more than just work—it is also a balance of learning to play. Just because we have grown up, it doesn't mean we can't still play and have fun.

What are you going to try? Once you start to experiment, you may learn even more about yourself. Perhaps you will find hidden gifts or talents.

Exercise

Again I am thankful to Irena, as she got me moving again. She had a friend who taught yoga, but I was reluctant to try it because of what other people were saying. The truth is, I appreciated the slow exercise and that it was making me use my muscles again. After lying in bed for such a long time, my body had lost so much muscle strength.

During this time, I learned how to quiet my mind and how to *be still*. My practice was different from how others may do it. My time was spent in continuous prayer in the presence of God. This was the start of me getting back to a place where I was moving my body and gaining more strength. Yoga taught me how to hold my peace by being still.

Exercise is so important, as we all need to be moving to keep the body healthy. Once I was in better shape, I joined a gym for a short time, but in truth, I do better in my home. So I went back to DVDs in the comfort of my own home, and began to feel the muscle growing stronger every day.

How are you doing when it comes to exercise? Are you moving every day? Friends, start somewhere. If you have an alignment or an illness stopping you from exercise, then start with something you can handle—perhaps just walking on the spot in the comfort of your living room while watching a TV program. Start getting up during the commercials and resting in between. Once you have built up your strength, you will be walking through a whole program. Before you know it, you will be outside taking in the fresh air and the colours of healing all around you in nature. Some of you may prefer to just dance in your living room or head out to the gym. Start wherever you are comfortable and be prepared to feel better and better every day—one step at a time.

Deception from Darkness
Chapter Seven

O ften we take far too much for granted in life, and sadly this often includes the precious people we love the most. I will never be able to thank my daughter and husband enough for standing by my side through our journey of illness and financial loss. When illness comes along, it can take much more than just our health. It also has the power to destroy families if we aren't careful.

In a world that is badly out of balance, we can see how even technology is destroying relationships and families. Friends, we need to be on guard; watch for these signs and recognize what is not from God. We all know there is darkness in this world. We need to be ready to defend and protect our lives and those whom we love the most. The Word says, *"Stay alert! Watch out for your great enemy, the devil. He prowls around like a roaring lion, looking for someone to devour. Stand firm against him, and be strong in your faith"* (1 Peter 5:8–9). We must stay focused on the light of God, or the darkness will devour us.

Have you ever noticed how technology is destroying lives? Today, more than ever, people are losing relationships because of these devices. I am not saying everything about technological devices is bad, because they do help us stay connected with people far away, and are very helpful in many ways. But when you allow this to get out of *balance*, it opens the door for darkness to work.

Look around you and watch people. I am amazed at how many people are in restaurants with their families and both parents are on their phones, missing the blessing of being present with their children. This is a time in your life you can't get back. Your children grow up quickly, so enjoy the precious moments of time with them. What about all the husbands and wives who can't seem to communicate anymore, but are busy having conversations with someone outside of the home? Rather than leaving the home to meet someone in secret, inappropriate relationships are now being created from within the home. People feel it isn't cheating on their spouse, but in truth it's an emotional disconnection. That disconnection is when the cheating begins—you have given your emotions to another person. This only moves you farther away from your spouse and closer to the person you are talking with.

Friends, children today are losing communication skills because it's much easier to text than to actually say something face to face. In truth, they are hiding behind the screen of their device. I believe many of the conversations and pictures people are sharing would not exist if it wasn't so easy.

I remember visiting years ago with an elderly man whom I respected a great deal. I used to love visiting with him, as he always shared such wisdom. One day he said these words which have stayed with me: "You know, people think we have come so far. Just look around you and you will see what I am talking about. The other day I went for a walk and I saw a group of young kids out in the park where I was walking among the trees. It was so sad—they were all on their phones, missing this precious moment in nature and the time with one another. None of them were able to see anything or hear anything because their phones had their minds preoccupied and distracted. The truth is, we are further away from one another than ever. When will people wake up?"

Here is some food to ponder. I am a visual person and I see things symbolically. This was something shared with me, and I challenge you to think about it for yourself. What about the logo for Apple? In the Garden of Eden, deception came to Adam and Eve through the cleverness of the enemy, who simply put doubt into their minds. They fell for the deception and took a bite out of the apple. We are descended from these two people. So are we being deceived too?

As I was writing this, I saw a program on TV where a whole shipment of free computers was being donated to a school. The teachers and students were all jumping up and down with excitement. I almost didn't put this in the book, because my first thought was how wonderful it was that this big computer company was donating all these gifts. In truth, though, maybe it is part of the deception. The world is so out of balance due to technology, as we can't live without all of our conveniences. But those conveniences come with a price tag on our children's health and ours as well. Studies show that more depression and anxiety exist today. Doctors believe it is technology and social media that has caused this increase in numbers of people suffering.

However, in 2020 when the coronavirus hit our world, technology was a hidden blessing to many of us. Sometimes God can use for good the very thing the enemy plans to destroy people's lives with. Just think about how technology allowed us to still connect with our families and loved ones at such a dark time. Many people still gathered as a church family, and even more, people became receptive to learn and hear more about faith from those who became bolder in sharing their hearts with those they love. I love seeing the good come out of things that are meant to hurt people. This has been a larger blessing to those who don't know Jesus, and it was a huge wakeup call for all believers.

Friends, we know that balance is the key to everything in life, so try to be mindful and really pay attention. Is your device a problem for you? Can you go a few days without it, or even a few hours? Perhaps that is the problem. If this is something you feel is a concern for you, what can you do to balance this behaviour? You can start by monitoring how much time you are actually spending on your device. It will truly amaze you. What may seem like five minutes can quickly turn into half an hour. If you feel life is too busy and you have no time, perhaps this will help reveal where some of your time is going. If you have good self-control, start by setting times when you will allow yourself to check your phone. For example, at 9 a.m., 12 p.m., and 4 p.m. Another great idea is to give yourself a time limit each time you use your device. When you log on your device, set your alarm for the set amount of time you are willing to spend—perhaps ten minutes. By simply making these small changes, you will be the one in control, and that gives you greater power. Remember, balance is everything.

There are many things around that deceive all of us, and many Christians are being misled by following the ways of the world. Remember, friends, the best way to learn if you are being misled is to stay close to God every day and keep soaking up His Word. If you want to discern things, always test them with the Word. To discern what is right and wrong and see who is speaking as a false prophet, you need to test it.

Dear friends, do not believe everyone who claims to speak by the Spirit. You must test them to see if the spirit they have comes from God. For there are many false prophets in the world. This is how we know if they have the Spirit of God: If a person claiming to be a prophet acknowledges that Jesus

Christ came in a real body, that person has the Spirit of God. But if someone claims to be a prophet and does not acknowledge the truth about Jesus that person is not from God. Such a person has the spirit of Antichrist, which you heard is coming into the world and indeed is already here.

But you belong to God, my dear children. You have already won a victory over those people, because the Spirit who lives in you is greater than the spirit who lives in the world. Those people belong to this world, so they speak from the world's viewpoint, and the world listens to them. But we belong to God, and those who know God listen to us. If they do not belong to God, they do not listen to us. That is how we know if someone has the Spirit of truth or the Spirit of deception.

—1 John 4:1–6

I believe it's important to share this next story, which I haven't told many people before because it seemed so *unbelievable*. Some people may think it's way out there, but I believe there are others who have fallen for the kind of deception I'll describe shortly. The lie can become a stronghold in their lives, stopping them from being used in a powerful way for God to help others. I share this to show others how the enemy can take hold of a person at a very young age and plant lies in their minds to control them.

Somehow in my early childhood, I developed the suspicion that I might have been adopted. Maybe you have experienced a similar belief. From the time we are born until about the age of six, we are like sponges, absorbing everything we see and hear. I am not sure why I believed this lie about myself— perhaps it was something I heard as a little girl from someone. But those words became a part of me trapped in my mind, and they stayed with me my whole life until I put an end to it.

When I used to ask my parents if I had been adopted—which I did frequently—they would make light of the question and just say, "How could you be adopted when you look so much like your sisters?" I don't know where this idea ultimately came from, but I felt like I was different from my siblings.

Around the time I fell ill, this thought came back in my life, only more strongly than ever before. It was actually tormenting me. I spoke about it with a couple of people, but their responses only reinforced my suspicion. This was when I began to test the spirits with the truth in the Bible. Anything we are believing and focusing our minds on becomes our reality. I believe many people have doors not of God that need to be closed, but evil lies are trying to keep them open.

One day the thought came to my mind: instead of wondering and giving any more energy to this subject, why not ask again? Why not go right to the source? I went to my mother and told her I needed to put something completely out of my mind for good. I no longer wanted this door of doubt left open—not even a crack. It needed to be closed for good with the truth.

Sometimes, the lie we believe and the doubt we have are all it takes to make a lie feel real. I remember before asking my mother the question, I had prepared myself to learn something potentially very difficult. The truth was, I was ready for anything, and believed that no matter what the answer was, I would be able to move forward with no more deception in my life.

That day, I simply asked the question. "When I was young, I used to ask you if I was adopted, and it was kinda a running joke because I looked so much like my family. Today, I am asking for 100% honesty so I can put this lie to bed. Give it to me straight. Was I perhaps given to you to be raised by someone else within our family tree?"

I remember the look on my mom's face. She was surprised and hurt all at the same time. How could I believe such a lie? But that is how the enemy works in a person's mind. I have no regrets over asking the question, because it gave me an unbelievable peace back that had been taken from me many years ago. The enemy likes to get a hold of people to try and take them off their God-given path.

I remember thinking I would have been okay if she responded, "Yes you were," because then Ted and I would have had one more thing in common. My husband was adopted, and I thought maybe our story would have been similar. For any of you out there that are adopted, I want to leave you with this amazing thought. When two people decide to have a child, they are blessed by getting what God gives them. For any of you out there that are adopted, though, you are extra special because you were chosen. Your parents got to choose you for themselves. Now, I think that is pretty powerful!

I often think of the Family of God. That's how we are. We are chosen by God: before we even knew Him, He chose us! He loves us. Pretty awesome, don't you think? *"But you are not like that, for you are a chosen people. You are royal priests, a holy nation, God's very own possession. As a result, you can show others the goodness of God, for he called you out of the darkness into his wonderful light"* (1 Peter 2:9).

I will always be so very grateful to my mom, for without her I wouldn't be here on this amazing journey. Motherhood can be a tough job at times, and it's one I have come to appreciate even more since I became a momma myself. Mom, I am thankful for your understanding and patience with me. It is really the love of our mothers that goes without saying. Thanks, Mom, for being you and loving me. I may not say it often enough, but I love you.

I encourage all of you out there to tell your kids often how much they are loved. It's something we all need to hear more during our lives.

Is there some lie you were told as a child that has held you captive for many years? The truth will set you free—so ask for what you need, and don't let deception and darkness hold you in bondage any longer. When we approach people with tough questions and *do it in love*, it becomes *a gift of freedom.* We are no longer victims, but rather we move into victory! I hope that by sharing these small stories, it will shed light on how easily we can be taken off course throughout our lives if we are not careful and alert. The darkness wants to destroy us, but when we live in the light, nothing can harm us. All thanks to God!

I am so thankful for the times when God has protected me from the deception that happens all too easily. There was a time back in 2014 when I was supposed to be going to a ladies' conference, but I felt God was asking me to go north alone and spend my time with Him. I knew there would be drinking back in the hotel room. At that time, I was really struggling with my pain and didn't want to fall back into addiction.

I am sharing this with you because many times we don't always recognize when the enemy is trying to hurt us. Sometimes he will attack us through people or through circumstances in order to break us. In some cases, we are even used unknowingly, and unfortunately we have probably taken others off course too. Our words contain power, and we have to be very careful how we use them so that we don't cause another person to fall.

When I was getting ready to head north to be alone in His presence, I had to make a few quick stops before I left. At one of the stops, I was so discouraged. The person I'd seen had made the suggestion that when I got to the cottage, I should kick back and have a few glasses of wine. I couldn't get to my car quickly enough, and the tears began to fall down my cheeks. How could the people I love suggest wine when I hadn't had a drink in over three years? The very things I was trying to avoid were now being suggested to me.

As I drove up the highway, I had to pull over as I could no longer see the road from all the tears. I called my sister Darlene and told her what had happened. She said a prayer with me and reminded me "God is your strength."

I highly encourage you to get a prayer partner for the times you can't pray for yourself, and be prepared to listen to the Spirit when He lays someone on your heart. Many of us miss important messages from the Spirit, but we can be used to help others if we are listening. Have you ever had this happen to you before? You are busy doing something and you suddenly think of someone—*I should call that person*—but the moment passes and before you know it, a week rolls by and you still haven't called them.

Quite often the Spirit will just lightly "tap us on the shoulder," letting us know that someone needs to hear from us. Perhaps they need some prayers for encouragement, and we miss the calling because we are too distracted with life. There have been many times when the Spirit has had me pull over in my car to call someone right then and there. As it turned out, they needed something and were blown away that the call came when they needed it most.

That's how God works through us. It takes time to hear His voice, and I've missed so many opportunities in the past. I remember one time when I thought of a person we had helped out years earlier and stayed in contact with. That day I felt I needed to call him, but life got busy and I put it off. I remember calling him a week later to the day, because I received a much more intense "tap on the shoulder" telling me to call him. I learned he had been in a bad accident. That's when he could have used me the most—not a week later!

Back to my weekend retreat at the cottage with God. When I arrived there and unloaded my cooler and guitar from the car, I would understand the prayer that my sister had prayed with me on the side of the road a little better. When I opened the fridge door to put the groceries away, there was a bottle of red wine sitting on the second shelf looking at me.

I looked up and said, "You have got to be kidding me!"

"Go ahead, Sam—you can drink the whole bottle and no one will see you. Go ahead, it's okay," I heard a voice say.

But then I heard God's voice in my heart: "Don't do it, Sam. You don't want to fall into addiction again."

As soon as this happened, I took the bottle outside to the shed and told myself, "Out of sight, out of mind." I would not be broken, no matter how hard things were getting!

What would have happened to me if I had not stopped and had someone pray with me to renew my strength? I believe my story would be very different than it is today, and I don't believe I would be writing this. So always remember—when we take our prayers and petitions to the Lord, He gives us everything we need. I believe God knew what was best for me when He asked me to give alcohol up before Lyme disease arrived on my doorstep. If I hadn't given it to Him, I know it would have been my way of coping with the pain. Thank God I was listening. I could have lost more than my wine—I could have lost my family, the most precious and priceless gift I have.

I want to share something else with you, because I believe many of us are deceived even about ourselves. Over the years of growing, learning, and changing to be the best version of myself, I have come to see things so much differently. As I share this idea, I hope it will shed light for you as well. You know the times you grow impatient with people or they frustrate you or even make you downright angry? I started another mission to help me understand what it was I was seeing in other people.

The truth is, the eyes are the gateway to a person's soul. When something irritates me or causes me to lose my peace when I am around others, I will go to a mirror and look at myself. Looking into my own eyes, I ask God to show me what it is that I see in them that I cannot see in myself. Most times He shows me quickly, and I am so grateful for the conviction as it shows me the truth in my own life. What I am aware of in myself brings even greater changes.

Here is a question for you. Have you been feeling that little tap on your shoulder lately, telling you that something needs to change? Maybe you have been feeling it for a while, but like me, you didn't want to acknowledge it because you knew it was going to involve some work on your part. I believe the fear of the unknown is stopping many people. Change is difficult, and it frightens people. It's much easier to stay in the place you are because it's familiar and comfortable. The truth is, God wants so much more for you.

I love how many words in the English language have hidden words within them that build us up even more. Just think about the word *encouragement*. Right there in that very word is the word you need to keep moving forward. *Courage!*

If you are feeling lost or need guidance about something, ask friends and family to start praying for you. Look up and ask for wisdom on how to move forward. I believe far too many people are caught in that place of being the victim, which is not any way to live. My prayer is for you to see that the decision you make today will move you into victory. It all begins with making the right choices and taking the right path.

Don't be afraid, for I am with you. Don't be discouraged, for I am your God. I will strengthen you and help you. I will hold you up with my victorious right hand.

—Isaiah 41:10

...even there your hand will guide me, and your strength will support me.

—Psalm 139:10

Your word is a lamp to guide my feet and a light for my path.

—Psalm 119:105

Resources
Chapter Eight

We have all had times in our lives when our resources have caused stress or concerns in our lives (with or without illness on our doorsteps). For Ted and me, coming up against Lyme disease with no treatment available in Canada, no disability benefits or financial resources to help with the treatment, we were really embarking on the hardest test of all.

During this journey, our long-time friends Steve and Melissa held a garage sale, with all proceeds coming to us. They will never know how greatly we appreciated this kindness, and we will never forget it. The money went towards my monthly treatment, and a niece of mine also started a GoFundMe to help raise funds. Ted and I really struggled to accept these resources, as we had sold our home and were truly worried what people would think of us for asking for help.

I remember visiting with my pastor, and he shared these words with me: "There are people who want to help you, and this is one way they can—that's how God works through people." Although this made it a little easier to accept the help, it still did not come easily for us. We were raised believing you never ask for help, and if you borrow money, you always have to pay it back with interest.

I believe many things we adults struggle with come from the way we were raised. I am in no way saying what my mom and dad taught me is wrong, but I do believe we also need to learn how to accept help. It's all about giving and receiving with balance. We don't want to be that person who takes and never gives. At the same time, we shouldn't always be a giver without ever receiving. Everything in life is good when we use balance.

When April set up the GoFundMe, it was used for my monthly treatment. We will always be so grateful to everyone who came to help us in our hour of need. I truly believe with all my heart that it's not the amount that counts as much as the heart that is helping. We give out of love. Eventually, we decided to shut it down and thought we could keep selling our material possessions, as we needed more resources. We hoped that we wouldn't lose everything we had worked so hard for. In the Bible, we know it says that the root of all evil is the love of money. It's not money itself but the *love* of money that causes so many problems for people.

I share this because for many of us, money is a stronghold, whether you are blessed with abundance or you struggle to make ends meet. The ones who have much are afraid to lose what they have, and the ones who have little are afraid they won't have enough. So whether it is great or little, we see fear.

Often we adapt our family's beliefs about money. Whatever we grow up hearing and seeing about money becomes our reality as well. Many times, it's just a cycle and pattern that leads into worry and frustration around the subject. If you grew up hearing your parents say they never had enough money, then you are going to believe money is a hard thing to have and to keep. Perhaps you heard a lot of arguments over finances, and now you find this is an area of conflict in your own life today. If you grew up where all you heard was "I have to work so I will have money," you probably work far too much because that's what you heard and believe to be true for you as well.

Again, money is all about balance. One thing is true—money needs to keep moving. If we stop the flow of it in our own lives, it can't come back to us. If we are always trying to have more and more for ourselves but never learn to share and serve with our resources, again it will be hard to see it come back into our lives.

This may sound unbelievable to many, but I am so glad that God has allowed Ted and me to journey with a disease that has no funding, because the experience has taught us something far greater. When you have to endure hardships like other people, you understand them better and can relate more easily with their pain.

This disease has taken Ted and me down some hard roads when it comes to finances. We had to learn to live on one income with a hefty financial burden imposed by my monthly treatment. When I had to quit work, we quickly learned that we needed to downsize or we'd go even deeper into debt. After almost a year of lost income (not knowing how long I might be off), we decided to sell our home and buy a small mobile home, which we felt we could manage more easily. We had a place all lined up with the closing date only two weeks away when the deal fell through. Now we had two weeks to find a home. This was stress we didn't need in our life—especially not while I was ill.

The amazing part about this story is that God already had a place for us. I remember my father telling me that I should call the owner of the farm we had once owned to see if they would let us move in. At that time, the house had been sitting empty, and this became an answered prayer for us. This family has been a true gift from above. We moved in right away and are still renting this home as of 2020.

I was blown out of the water! I believed then that I was coming home to my childhood home for a reason. I believed my life would end where it had started. I had come full circle in the story of my life, or so I thought. But once I got home, I began to realize God had brought me home to teach me even greater lessons about how things are passed down through the generations (which I hope I can share in another book someday). The healing that I needed would begin here so that my life could take me further into my greater purpose.

Back in 2012, my mom and dad were at our home for dinner. This was the winter before I fell ill. Dad shared some words with me, and it wasn't until after he passed that I really thought about them. I believe people often share wisdom that we miss, only to understand it later.

That evening at dinner, he said these words: "Why don't you sell your home now so that you won't have to work so hard? You could go rent a home and keep your cottage. You could even go rent our old farmhouse from the new owners."

I told my dad, "Yes, that is the plan, but we can't swing it yet. There's no way we could ever afford to live in the old farmhouse. I need to keep working for at least another five years."

"I don't think you can keep working as hard as you are now without burning out," he replied.

Dad was right about two things: I did burn out, and—how bizarre!—the very place he told me we should go to live was where we later ended up. God does work in mysterious and miraculous ways. Many times, others may be saying words we should really be listening to.

Trusting when you don't understand His ways is the largest test of them all—especially when it comes to finances. In the human realm, it's hard to understand how things could possibly work out when it comes to money or lack of it. But it amazes me how God works everything together in your time of need.

We were attending a wedding one September weekend. I had paid all our bills on Friday, leaving us with only a hundred dollars left in our account. That day, I received a phone call from a sister from our church. She asked if I would be at the wedding the following day, as she had something to give me. I already knew it would be a gift from God, but I had no idea what it was. I love it when people are told by God to do something and they are obedient to Him; otherwise, I wouldn't have received this valuable message.

That Saturday morning, after I wrote a cheque for the wedding gift our balance was left at zero. I had just finished a devotion that said God takes care of you, even right down to your last penny. When I arrived at the wedding, my friend came running up to me to share a story about how God had taken her for a walk earlier that week. While she was out walking, she heard Him tell her to watch for some money, which she found to be rather a strange request—but she followed His instructions. As she walked along, she found a penny, and was so excited because God had blessed her with this special gift. As the week went on, she said my face kept coming into her mind, and she was getting rather frustrated because she felt she was to give me this special penny. In obedience, she handed me the penny.

When I checked the year on the penny it was 2010, which had a special meaning to me, and I smiled because I knew God had sent me a message. It was this: *"Don't worry about anything; I see you and all the things you are going through, and it will all work out. Be patient and trust Me."*

We experience things that don't make sense in the human realm, but that's how I know it's God—because it is *miraculous*. I have had times where I am paying our bills, and on paper we shouldn't have any resources left or at most there should be very little in our account, but the balance shows something different. I have gone back trying to find where the money came from without being able find a trace. How does that work? Only God can make things like that happen, and I am always in awe of Him when He does.

When we are waiting for things to happen, it can feel like it's taking forever—but with God, His timing is perfect, even if we can't understand it. He has a special purpose for everything, and He will work it all out for the good of everyone around us.

What is it you need more trust for? Perhaps it's that relationship that seems to be dying because of your resources or interference from another person. Maybe it's your own health or that of someone you love. You don't think you have the resources—well, you need to try something different. Don't let the enemy attack you in the weakest areas of your life. Instead, let God fight your battles. *Where there is a will, there is a way!* Be encouraged.

I believe that when we take time to reflect, we start to see that in most cases the things we are worrying about are just wasting our energy and time. In the end, have you ever gone hungry? Have you ever been homeless? Have you ever been without clothing? The truth is, God is always providing, just like He provides for the birds outside. If He takes care of the birds and animals, why can't we trust Him to take good care of us too? Believe His Word.

One thing I like to do that builds my trust in God is to put up cards with scriptures of affirmation where I will see them every day. This is the same idea as the vision board, but these are simple reminders to help you stay focused. When you read the words often, you begin to believe what you are hearing, especially if you say them in your own voice. So keep them in sight and speak those words over your life every day. You will be amazed at how much better you begin to Trust Him.

For example, you could write:

I know that God is working on my finances,
and He will make everything possible.

God loves me and will never leave nor forsake me.

I trust you, Jesus!

I know good things are happening in my life
and God will restore what I have lost.

God's healing power is working in my life every day.
I am getting better and better.

Another wonderful idea is to keep a remembrance box. When something wonderful happens and you witness God providing something for you, write about it. Write down what happened, and put a date on the paper. I always like to write a note of thanks on the sheet, too. When you find you are going through a dry time in your life, pull out a memory to remind yourself how good God is and that He always provides at the perfect time.

Here is another beautiful thing that you can also do. Have a coin jar and start with the decision that with what you save in this jar, you are going to sew some good seeds. I heard this once from a friend whose father said, "If you take good care of your coins, the bills will take care of themselves." The truth is, you may see your change as nothing but change, but through this exercise, you will see the loose coins become the *"change"* you want to see in your life. In the Bible, there is a story about a woman who gave all she had, which was a single coin. Others who had much may have given more, but it wasn't all they had. Her gift was of greater value because she gave all she had with all her heart.

Never underestimate what you can give, because we all have something to offer. Try this: save your change for the next month. At the end of the month, look for ways to bless someone. Perhaps your jar will have $8.oo at the end of the month. You could decide to buy coffee for four people, or treat someone to lunch, or simply buy some small items to bless others with. The more you do for others, the more you will be blessed. It really does get exciting, because you will start to see a return of blessings in your life. They may not always come back as resources, but they could return to you in a different way. We don't give to receive, but rather because a giving heart is a happy heart. You will begin to see more joy released into your own life because you are sowing seeds. We can't get a harvest without planting. So get excited—know that God sees all the small things you are doing, and He is pleased.

Jesus looked at them intently and said, "Humanly speaking, it is impossible. But with God everything is possible."

—**Matthew 19:26**

That is why I tell you not to worry about everyday life—whether you have enough food and drink, or enough clothes to wear. Isn't life more than food, and your body more than clothing? Look at the birds. They don't plant or harvest or store food in barns, for your heavenly Father feeds them. And aren't you far more valuable to him than they are? Can all your worries add a single moment to your life?

And why worry about your clothing? Look at the lilies of the field and how they grow. They don't work or make their clothing...

—**Matthew 6:25–28**

The Healing of Nature
Chapter Nine

When I started the quest of searching for my healing, I was very blessed to have lots of quiet time up north at our cottage. I believe our bodies cannot receive healing if the environment we are in is filled with stress or negative emotions. It took me a long time to learn that if I was around people who gossiped a lot, it only hurt my spirit. It really seemed to affect me more during my illness. Whatever it is, the environment that you allow yourself to be in will affect you. Everything you see and hear is working in you—more than you realize. It can begin to rub off on you like a disease. Healing needs a good environment with peace surrounding you.

I can remember years earlier, before I fell ill, wishing I could take time from work to go north with our daughter Ashley for an extended amount of time. That was something I really wanted to do, whether she was in public school or high school or college—to spend quality time alone with her. But it seemed we were never in a financial place that we could swing it.

Life is so amazing: how your dreams come true, only in a different way. But they still did come true! To be honest, I believe we allow our resources to take away from our dreams. The truth is, we were not in any better position financially—in fact, things were even more difficult. But it was my perspective that had been changed through my illness. While Ashley completed her summer college co-op, she lived at the cottage with me. It was a great season, and I will always cherish the time we shared together.

When I first fell ill, for two summers I was basically in bed all the time. I really had no life. People at the cottage were wondering where I had disappeared to. So when I was able to stay up north and begin the healing process, I was beyond grateful. I have been blessed with a precious gift that many do not get. *Time.* I do believe this has been the greatest asset in healing—allowing myself the time I needed to heal. I am truly thankful that Ted and Ashley were always so supportive of this. We all heal differently, but I do believe there is nothing better than being one with nature and surrounded by God's amazing power.

There are many benefits from being out in nature, and I truly embraced this time to soak in every ounce of healing I could. People do not realize that healing comes through our five senses and everything has healing power in it.

The colours you surround yourself with give you healing. Everything from the different shades of green in the trees, the sun, the blue skies, flowers, birds, and water.

Every sound you hear releases more healing. The sounds of the birds, the wind blowing through the trees, the snap and popping of a campfire, chipmunks, squirrels, and the sounds of water.

Each smell you take in, everything you touch and taste has healing properties in it. Is it any wonder there is so much healing around us when we know who created it all? Do you know that feeling of walking through freshly cut grass in your bare feet, or the sensation of sand between your toes? It's funny when you think about life. Some people will pay their hard-earned resources to replace what is free outside just to do it indoors. Take time, friends, to embrace this amazing creation that was given to you for your enjoyment.

It seemed every summer I was being amazed more and more with many revelations, and many moments when I knew my body, mind, and spirit were all healing. I spent my summer studying God's word, playing guitar, kayaking, lighting lots of campfires, playing in the water, and taking lots of hikes, trying to build my physical strength back up. I really focused on healthy eating during this time too. Another thing I am so grateful for: we have a waterfall not far from our cottage, so I spent a great deal of time there. The sound of the running water did wonders for my body, as well as for my spiritual ears and eyes, helping me understand things I once didn't. Again, it all involves frequencies that produce healing.

I can remember one day when I had the desire to walk along the river. I have no idea why, but I put my water shoes on and began to walk down the centre of the river. As I was making my way through the water, I just soaked in the sights, sounds, and touch of liquid against my legs. As I got closer to the falls, my heart began to race. I remember at one point I stopped and my feet weren't sure where to go, so I just stood there for a moment.

In life, we can feel like we are losing our footing and we just stop. We get stuck, unable to move forward. Sometimes we wander off to the left or to the right because an obstacle makes it too hard to go forward. That day, my obstacle was the falls ahead. Uncertain of the ground below me, I went to the right to test out the ground below the water. It was solid and secure, so I made my way out of the river.

I believe every day we can find lessons in nature, but we miss the message because of fear and distractions. My summer north has given me so many quiet messages through the water, a sunrise or sunset, the clouds, or even a campfire. I remember one time when it was almost dark and I felt prompted to go down to the river and just set my feet in the water at the falls. I wasn't overly excited as it was turning dark, but I knew I was to go—so off I went. I can remember just sitting there and feeling this amazing peace wash over me. I knew something wonderful was coming, but again I was not sure when or what.

Three days later, I received a call from my friend Irena, just checking in to see if it was okay for her to come for a visit to the cottage. Honestly, I was trying to cancel this visit, as I was still struggling with my strength and didn't feel like company. During the conversation, she said she would be up and that we should go to the waterfall. Irena loves waterfalls and she was the one to encourage me to spend lots of time near them. The day she came, we spent some time swimming in the water hole and then she told me to lay back into the water. As I lay there floating, she began to do reflexology on my feet. I had my ears under the water, just allowing the sounds of the pounding water to resonate throughout my body. I remember that afternoon being beautiful, with the gorgeous bright sun beating down on us and the big open blue sky all around us.

During this experience, I had my eyes closed, but I knew something was happening to my body. It felt like a brilliant bright light moving through my body with a warming sensation that tingled through me. I felt as if I was smiling from within, and I was filled with unbelievable joy and warmth. When we got back to the cottage to have lunch, I shared with Irena that I felt like something had happened to me and she said she could tell by the way I was responding. I believe I was able to receive it because I really wanted to. I believe God brought me this wonderful experience because three days earlier, I had been obedient to what He was asking of me.

It reminds me of the story in the Bible of the man who lay beside the pool at Bethesda.

*Inside the city, near the Sheep Gate, was the pool of Bethes-
da, with five covered porches. Crowds of sick people—blind,
lame, or paralyzed—lay on the porches. One of the men lying
there had been sick for thirty-eight years. When Jesus saw
him and knew he had been ill for a long time, he asked him,
"Would you like to get well?"*

*"I can't, sir," the sick man said, "for I have no one to
put me into the pool when the water bubbles up. Someone else
always gets there ahead of me."*

*Jesus told him, "Stand up, pick up your mat, and
walk!"*

*Instantly, the man was healed! He rolled up his sleep-
ing mat and began walking!*

—John 5:2–9

I believe I was acting just like the man at the pool. When
Irena called, I looked for an excuse to keep her away, but God
was trying to bless me with a gift from Him. I believe we humans do this all the time. We find all kinds of excuses to stay
where we are instead of using our faith muscles to get up and
do something. Faith is an action word, and often it requires us
to do something for ourselves to release the power of God in
our lives. Does it always work that way? No, not always—but
we are taught to trust and have faith and be content with how
God plans to use our lives. I can tell you, the more I trust Him
and the more time I spend with Jesus, the more I am amazed.

One day a message came to me through a cloud. I was
sitting on my dock alone, praying about our finances and asking God what we should do. As I sat there in His presence, I
was admiring these five beautiful big puffy clouds that were
drifting slowly across the sky. One by one they disappeared
right before my eyes. In that instant, I knew I did not need to
worry about anything because God was on the job. It was as if

He spoke to my heart at that moment and all I heard was, "The debt is not yours. You did not cause it, but it will be taken care of." I was filled that day with an unbelievable peace, because it's not my burden to carry. He will make all things work out for good if I just keep trusting.

I often admire the beauty of the abundance in nature. There is nothing lacking. When you see all the beauty surrounding you, you truly have everything you need. I love looking at the glimmer of sparkles that shine off the surface of the lake from the sun. It just reminds me of God's amazing gifts, and that reflection just makes me see God's diamonds. They are everywhere!

Over the last few years, as my health has begun to come back to a better place, I've been amazed by other messages left for me. I started to find coins everywhere. One day while I was down at the waterfalls, I found a nickel hidden under the rock wall right after I had prayed about our resources. I love those moments, because it puts me right back to a place of trust. Everything started with that penny at the wedding. Next came this nickel, followed by a dime, and before long a quarter and then a loonie. I could see something beautiful happening as the next coin that arrived was a toonie. It seems the denominations were growing, and I just had to keep my eyes on Him.

One day, Ted and I were walking through a parking lot when a five-dollar bill flew through the air (there was a young boy walking across at the same time and Ted yelled for the little guy to grab the money). Not too long after that encounter, I was at a corn feast when a twenty-dollar bill flew right through the air and landed not far from my feet. I grabbed it and started hunting for the owner. I ended up leaving it at the front counter in case someone claimed their loss later that day.

I love how we all receive messages differently. We are all taught differently and we all see things differently, so why wouldn't we receive our messages the same way? Be encouraged—He does want to speak to you, however He can reach you. All you need is an open heart and to be willing to do what He asks of you.

I remember a young man I met who was talking about a wonderful canoe trip he had taken in the interior of a large park up north. As he told his story, I shared some of the amazing ways God had spoken to me through His beautiful creation.

He listened to what I wanted to say and replied, "Well, I don't know if I believe there is a God, but I had something similar happen to me while I was on this camping trip. We had just canoed through a large lake, and it was pouring with rain. It was truly a dark, damp morning, and all of a sudden it stopped raining instantly and I saw the most beautiful sunrise appear." He said it took his breath away because it was so beautiful, and he felt this amazing peace surrounding him.

I just smiled at this young man and said, "You, my friend, were having a beautiful moment with God." He didn't say anything, but I know it was true and I hope he remembers those words.

What do you do when you feel tired, exhausted, or down? Are you struggling with anxiety or depression? I suffered many years with debilitating anxiety. Whenever I had an anxiety attack, it would take so much strength from me. I would be down and out in bed with exhaustion for days. While it was happening, it felt like I was having a heart attack with major sweating and an inability to breathe. My doctor wanted to medicate me for this condition, but I told him I would find a way to cope with it on my own.

I learned quickly what my triggers were. I had to stay away from alcohol, tobacco, caffeine, and sugar. I needed to make time for myself to get outside as much as possible, as well as exercise deep breathing. Another important thing for me was to learn I couldn't rush—it just stole my peace and led me into anxiety. By making small changes in my life, I now make sure to leave early when I am going somewhere. This helps me to hold my peace. I now arrive early for appointments instead of rushing, so when I arrive I will have time to sit quietly and just be still.

My friends, I encourage you to take every moment you can and get outside. Make time to soak in the beauty around you. If you feel unwell, the outdoors are truly a great cure to rejuvenate and restore your strength. We can do so many things to help ourselves just by being flexible. Make time every day for fresh air, and take many deep breaths—they will allow more oxygen into your bloodstream, and they're great to help calm nerves when you are anxious or tired.

Give it a try right now. Stop and close your eyes. Take a deep breath and hold it for three seconds, then slowly exhale through your mouth. The more you learn to be at peace with yourself, the more you will reap a harvest, as this will be what will flow out of your life: peace, joy, comfort, and tranquility. Each breath is a gift, so take it all in and *enjoy* the journey.

Then he added, "Pay close attention to what you hear. The closer you listen, the more understanding you will be given—and you will receive even more. To those who listen to my teaching, more understanding will be given. But for those who are not listening, even what little understanding they have will be taken away from them."

—Mark 4:24–25

But when you pray, go away by yourself, shut the door behind you, and pray to your Father in private. Then your Father, who sees everything, will reward you.

—Matthew 6:6

But Jesus often withdrew to the wilderness for prayer.

—Luke 5:16

Put on your new nature, and be renewed as you learn to know your Creator and become like him.

—Colossians 3:10

Please Help Us

Chapter Ten

When you decide you really want to become well, it takes commitment, consistency, and resources. After I had done many different things to promote further healing in my life, particularly when it came to spiritual healing, I knew I had more work to do with my physical being as well. I truly had come a long way since the times I had laid in bed for hours every day, but one area that I was still struggling with was my energy level.

One day I had a call from a friend I had known for years from the previous town we lived in. She wondered if she could stop by to share something that she felt might help me as I continued to get my health back on track. I will never forget the day she came to visit me. I have learned over the past few years that we should always be willing to listen to people, as they may have the answers to our prayers.

My friend told me that she had been taking some natural supplements for about two years, and was seeing a huge benefit in her health. She wanted to share this in case it was the missing piece I had been searching for.

Before I begin to describe this amazing story, I want to make it very clear that Plexus Worldwide does not claim to treat or cure any disease—rather, it offers hope for people to live a life of health and happiness.

The day Stephanie came, she shared a great detail of information about a company called Plexus and their products, as well as giving me reading material with further information. When she left, I was a bit of a skeptic but I also knew I needed to do my own research and ask for guidance from above. Financial resources had often stopped me from trying things in the past, plus I'd tried so many other things that hadn't helped me. In my heart, I was struggling with the financial burden I had already put on our family.

When Ted came home, I shared all that Stephanie had told me about that day. Ted was on board right away—it was actually him that encouraged me to really think about it. One thing that made him so positive from the very beginning was the company's policy: if you are not one hundred percent happy with a product, you have sixty days to have a total refund. I will never forget Ted's words: "Why wouldn't you give it a try and see what it can do for you? You have nothing to lose. What if this is that missing key you have been waiting for?"

I am so glad I listened to Ted and was guided to try the products. After doing my research and learning more about these plant-based supplements, I truly came to believe they were my answered prayer. *"You cause the grass to grow for the livestock and plants for people to use"* (Psalm 104:14).

Before Stephanie arrived to share Plexus, I'd still been struggling with exhaustion quite badly. Ted and I had planned a trip up to Thunder Bay that September to go camping, and I was already preparing to cancel it. Thank goodness I didn't do that. After being on Plexus for only eight short weeks, I couldn't believe the difference in how I was feeling. I quickly realized that Ted needed these life-changing products too.

My new state of health gave me even greater hope that the trip would be possible, and it was. It was unbelievable. I felt like me again! For so many years, I'd been ill and unable to hike even short distances, but now I was away and living the dream vacation back in my favourite place—creation. Ted and I had two weeks of beautiful weather, hiking, camping, and lots of campfires. I was alive and well again. Some answered prayers won't happen unless you take that step of faith. I will always be grateful to Stephanie for sharing with me—otherwise, I could still be in bed. I will also always be grateful to Ted and his encouraging words that helped me take that step of faith for both of us.

When I started taking the supplements, I signed up as an Ambassador with the company, mainly to get the best possible price. I also knew I would receive some return on my own purchases to help with the monthly products Ted and I were utilizing. As time went on and I continued to heal, I now believed this was a gift that God had brought to our family to help bless other families too. There was a time I wondered how on earth we would be able to sustain taking these supplements, but again, I see it as investing in ourselves for a better future. I knew if God brought this to us, He would make a way—and He has.

Plexus is all about gut health. When you work on the gut and heal from the inside first, everything else in your life begins to get better. When we were created, we were designed to have eighty percent good gut bacteria and twenty percent bad, so when we die our bodies can decompose. But as time has gone on, because of chemicals in our foods, pesticides and sprays, environmental toxins, antibiotics, processed foods, and fast food, we have unfortunately been brought out of balance in our guts. Now we are moving in the opposite direction from how we were designed to run. Our gut is now more like twenty percent good and eighty percent bad. When we allow this imbalance to happen, it opens the door for disease and illness to the body.

As I shared earlier, my gut wall was basically destroyed by all the harsh antibiotics I had been on while doctors were trying to diagnose me. Now it would take me years to reverse all that damage, but at least I was on the right path for further healing. Believe me when I say that everyone needs to be on a good probiotic. It is the key to healing your gut.

One thing I found from taking these supplements was that not only was my body beginning to feel better, but my mind and spirit seemed happier too. I believe when we take care of the gut, it will also bring wonderful healing for those of us who struggle with anxiety and depression. As we start to feel better, we look forward to being more active, and we also begin to crave better foods. Going forward into the future, Ted and I want to continue to learn and to keep making wiser food choices. The good thing about a high-quality supplement is that it helps to give the body what it can't receive from even the healthiest foods. Our soil is badly depleted, so now the nutrients and vitamins don't appear naturally like they should.

One thing I never wanted to be labelled or remembered as is that "sick woman." I would much sooner be known as someone who shared hope with people, and Plexus was that missing piece in the puzzle. I shared earlier that I am a visual person and see things symbolically, and I remember when I saw the Plexus logo I interpreted it as "Please Help Us."

Plexus is more than a company. They are really like a family that cares about people and their wellbeing. I had the privilege of taking a trip to Florida in 2018 to a Plexus convention. It was pretty amazing, and it only convinced me even more that I was where I was meant to be. Through this trip, I made new friendships and met some wonderful people. This company has given me purpose and has even been teaching me more about myself. I have developed greater confidence and pushed myself out of my comfort zone when it comes to sharing with others. I believe more than ever that people are looking for something in life, and we all want to be loved and accepted. I know through this journey I am more certain of who I am, and I truly feel blessed to be surrounded with people that know this kind of love. I don't know of another company that is so encouraging. You work together, cheering each other on! That's the kind of place I want to be—where we help each other.

After I came home from that trip to Florida, I recognized that I needed to work on my own self-confidence—something that is built when you know who you are and who is in you. One way I did this was by creating a visual board with a picture from my trip to the convention. I put it in an 8 x 10 frame and surrounded my picture with all the words describing what I wanted to see in myself. Over time, it really has helped me to keep moving forward. Along with the vision board, I kept cards of affirmation to encourage myself. If you don't believe in yourself first, how can anyone else believe in you? If you want to see a change in the world, you have to be willing to work on yourself. If you want to help others, you have to be healthy enough to do the work that is your calling. Friends, please be encouraged as we end this chapter. Believe that you are worth the investment of time, energy, and resources to take good care of your temple. When you feel well, you are in a much better place to deal with life in general and those you love around you.

If you are interested in learning more, please go to mysite. plexusworldwide.ca/samcrow and begin your research. Before making any decisions in life, always pray and be led by the Spirit for your healing answers.

We can make our own plans, but the Lord determines our steps.

—Proverbs 16:9

If you need wisdom, ask our generous God, and he will give it to you.

—James 1:5

Your own ears will hear him. Right behind you a voice will say, "This is the way you should go," whether to the right or to the left.

—Isaiah 30:21

Human's Best Friend: Dog—God

Chapter Eleven

As we draw near to the end of our journey together, I want to close by sharing something I believe many people can relate to. Life is a journey and we are meant to live it looking forward, not backwards. It's like driving a car. The windshield is big and bright so you can take in everything ahead of you. The things you have experienced are what brought you to where you are today. They have made you who you are.

I like to take time every now and again to do some self-reflection. I think of it as having a peek in the rear-view mirror so I can see where I have come from. Most of the time, it helps me understand why some of the journey happened in the order it did, or why I had to go the way God was leading me. When I was younger, I wasn't being led by the Spirit like I am today so some of the consequences are of my own doing, but I do believe the lesson will be worth it. We may wish we didn't have to experience some of the consequences of making bad choices, but if we learn to stay on the narrow path because of what it has taught us, then it will become a blessing.

I began to understand many things I could not have understood before now—even things that happened way back in 1980 as an eleven-year-old girl at summer camp. Just recently, in 2016, Ted and I were out for a scenic drive near our cottage in Muskoka when we accidentally drove past that camp from all those years ago. Later, I would learn that it was no accident. Many things are predestined to happen—they happen for a reason.

I remember that day how I filled up with excitement at the thought of the memories I had made in this special place. Ted quickly turned our car around and we entered the long driveway to see if it would be okay if we walked around the property. I wondered if any old memories would surge into my mind. Once we pulled up to the main building, I met a young girl who welcomed us to the camp. I explained that I had come to this camp thirty-six years earlier, and wondered if she would mind if I took my husband for a walk around the property and took a few pictures.

This day would be the beginning of something that was going to set a lot of things in motion within me, and I didn't have a clue how much. At that time, I knew something special was happening, and even if I didn't understand it right at that moment, I would understand it one day. Usually, it makes more sense down the road when we look back. That's why I love to journal so much—because it's like a puzzle board that holds all the pieces we need to connect the dots.

I couldn't believe how emotional I became. It was like I was eleven years old again. The coolest part for me was remembering details that I had totally forgotten about. Being there in that moment made me reflect, and I was filled with so much of the joy that I remembered from that place. Perhaps that's why my cottage and the north country mean so much to me—because I connected with God there many years earlier.

Ted and I walked around for a good hour and I shared the details as my memory began to unlock. It would seem some keys were going to open more revelations. We wandered down to the water and I showed him where I had taken swimming and canoe lessons. We just stood at the water, admiring this amazing view.

I can remember thinking to myself, *Wow, this is amazing to be here thirty-six years later.* It also made me realize something else about time. Even though I hadn't been there for many years, it didn't seem like that long ago. I believe that more revelations will come from the visit, but maybe not until later in the future. Not much had changed in all that time, except the trees had filled in a lot. The sky was still the same, the water was the same, the sounds were the same, and this moment stood absolutely still in time.

As I stood looking up from the water to where the common room was, I realized you could no longer see the building due to all the growth that had taken place. It made me think about how different we look after the years go by—not just our physical appearance, but our insides, and more importantly, our *hearts.* How we keep growing, learning, and changing as life hands us all kinds of different challenges we have to go through.

I know I have said many times how I would never change the fact that I had to make this journey through Lyme disease. The lessons I have learned and continue to learn far outweigh the pain I had to go through. These are the times in our lives when we get a better perspective of who we are and what we are going to do with our lives.

I know that summer is one I will never forget as long as I live. Ted and I walked around and I showed him the property and the buildings—and believe it or not, I even remembered the cabin I stayed in. It was called "The Otter Slide." When I opened the door, my memory went back in time even more, triggered by the same smells from all those years ago. I never would have remembered that if we hadn't taken this walk. To be in a meaningful place—in person, physically—does something to a person's soul. When we were in the common room my mind took me back to the many times we would share food and songs. The laughter and joy I felt there. I often think of my camp counsellor, who will never realize how much she touched my life. I still have her picture and even carry a bookmark in my Bible that she gave me that summer in 1980.

Why was 1980 so significant for me? That was the summer I asked Jesus to come into my life—and I wouldn't realize it until all these years later that it was there He blessed me with a new name. When I went to camp, I went in as Sandra, and when I left, I was Sam. People often ask why I use the name Sam, and I explain that we had two Sandras in the cabin, so they gave me the name Sam to make it easier when they wanted our attention.

All these years later, the name Sam even has greater meaning for me. I believe I received a new name from God that week. When I grew up, I was disappointed that I wasn't named after someone special. The rest of my siblings had names chosen after someone in the family tree. I now realize I didn't need a special name because I would be given mine later, at the age of eleven. Now it brings me even more joy.

I recently found a letter that I now carry in my Bible. My youngest sister Christine was taking care of my dog Cindy while I was away, and I had sent her this letter to see how Cindy was doing. I remember the day I bought Cindy with my own money, and had the privilege of picking her out myself. It was only two years before I headed off to camp.

Cindy was my best friend, especially during my high school years. As everyone knows, school can be hard with peer pressure and stress. I can remember that many times when I'd had a rough day, Cindy was always ready and eager to give me a much-needed hug. Sometimes I would just hang on to her while the tears rolled down my cheeks. She truly was my best friend.

In 1980, I won a speaking contest at our school and was sent to the next competition in another school. I just felt honoured to be given the chance to share with more people. I wasn't very comfortable with public speaking, but looking back, perhaps I was being prepared for something in my adult life that I didn't think would be possible. I remember I got teased so badly for my topic because people didn't understand why I would choose what I did. My topic was on "My Best Friend, Cindy, My Dog."

I believe when we are sharing something we believe in with all our hearts, then it's worth the criticism or remarks we may have to endure. In the end, I have no regrets.

My dog Cindy taught me what real love is. She taught me to love unconditionally and to always see the best in people. I believe dogs are truly a gift from God on so many levels. They can raise our spirits just by being around us, and change a hard day into a beautiful one. They can look into your eyes, and you know they love you. They are faithful friends who are loyal and can teach us humans how to live. Truthfully, I am convinced dogs have short lives because they already know how to live and treat people. What a world we would live in if more people would just love as our dogs do. Many times, I have told people that one of the first questions I will be asking God when I arrive in Heaven is this: "Was it Your idea that dog should be spelled like God backwards?" I am being very honest—their qualities are very similar. They are all about *love*.

Maybe the love of your dog has taught you something, or perhaps your dog has helped you survive hard times. Our sweet Boston terrier, Sophie, got me through some of the darkest days of my life while battling Lyme disease. She was the friend that lay beside me in bed and comforted me just by her presence. Every time I looked into her eyes, all I could see was her bubbly personality, full of love and energy that encouraged me. She was a lifeline to keep me going! Anatole France has some very powerful words to ponder: "Until one has loved an animal, a part of one's soul remains unawakened."[1]

When I have opportunities to share my testimony in person, I like to do a visual where I start with a wine glass filled with dark liquid. As I continue my story, I pour more and more water into my glass. As I am doing this, the glass slowly overflows and the liquid becomes clearer, until eventually it's crystal clear.

The dark liquid represents my life before I would allow God to work in me. I was weighed down trying to cope with life, and was filled with worry, anxiety, fears, unforgiveness, pride, and addictions. Once I allowed God to pour into my cup, I began to feel His love, joy, peace, patience, goodness, faithfulness, kindness, gentleness, and self-control. Now my life looks like a glass that is crystal clear. I am lighter and my life is clearer than ever before. I have been filled with *His unbelievable joy and peace in a way I have never known before.*

Life is hard here, my friends, but more than anything Jesus wants you to know how much He loves you and that you are never alone. It really is very simple. He wants to be your best friend and give you the life He died for you to have—a life filled with more joy, more love, and more peace than you have ever known.

Take a few minutes and listen to a song by Matthew West called "The Story of Your Life." I have never met Matthew but I have been touched by his music, as well as Michael Tyrrell's music. I hope one day to thank each of these men for the music they shared with the world—the music that changed my life. To say thank you in person and deliver a hug to them would be a dream come true.

Friends, we are touched every day by people—some we have never even met and others we meet only once—but something they share with us leaves an impression on us. There are others who leave our life only to return many years later, or we may be blessed to have had one person who has stood by us through the test of time.

As you finish this book, know that you have that same power to offer to the world. You can be a part of that ripple effect—a hope healer. A person who helps others find their way to move into a life they will truly love. We can all choose what legacy we want to leave the world—and it does start with you. In closing, I have only two questions for you:

Are you tired of how you are living? Do you want a different life?

If your answer to these questions is yes, I encourage you to ask Jesus to come into your life right now and begin the amazing journey that never ends. You will begin living your life for eternity today. This is your life, and it is only between you and Jesus. In the comfort of your own home, you can say these words to Him and He will come.

Jesus, I invite You now into my heart to guide my life in truth and change me. Forgive me for my past mistakes and help me to forgive those who have hurt me. I pray that with Your help I can turn away from the things that are hurting me and making my life more difficult. I want to heal, and I thank You that You love me right now unconditionally.

Jesus, take the wheel of my life and guide me with Your Holy Spirit in all that I say and do. I want my life to display Your love to everyone I meet. I thank You for the free gift of salvation You have given me today. I believe in God the Father, Jesus the Son, and the Holy Spirit. I am your child. Amen

Date: _____

Be sure to share this special moment in your life with your family and friends. Blessings and love as you begin a new life. It's going to be awesome! To nurture your relationship with Jesus, make sure you spend time in *His Word*, the Bible, and spend time in His presence every day.

But the Holy Spirit produces this kind of fruit in our lives; love, joy, peace, patience, kindness, goodness, faithfulness, gentleness, and self-control. There is no law against these things!

—Galatians 5:22–23

The Journey Continues...

Life is a journey, not a race. We are meant to take it one day at a time and to appreciate the journey for the lessons it is teaching us. I get excited to see where our family is heading, and I look forward to each new adventure. This is just part of the trip on our way home, with better days yet to come. I know I still have much to learn and many things to rise above, but it's going to be awesome if I keep my eyes focused upward....

Contact Information and Resource List

Here is a list of contacts if you desire to research more for yourselves. Blessings and healing in your journey ahead.

Contact me:

samcrowloveyourlife@gmail.com

Facebook:

lovestartstoday.ca
(https://www.facebook.com/lovestartstoday25/)

samcrowloveyourlife
(https://www.facebook.com/samcrowloveyourlife/)

Instagram:

@samcrowloveyourlife
(https://www.instagram.com/samcrowloveyourlife/?hl=en)

More resources:

Plexus Worldwide – Sandra (Sam) Crow
mysite.plexusworldwide.ca/samcrow

Word Alive Press
if you wish to order additional copies of this book
https://word-alive-press-bookstore.myshopify.com/

Wholetones: The Sound of Healing – Michael S. Tyrrell
home.wholetones.com

Bioreflex Therapies International – Irena Mariola Pawul
mlpawul@gmail.com

Dr. Michael Yarish at the Lakeside Clinic Center
for Integrated Medicine
www.thelakesideclinic.com

Looking for a Bible that is easy to understand? Try *Application Study Bible, New Living Translation*, second edition.

Also by the Author:

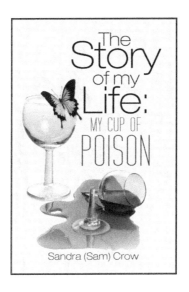

The Story of My Life: My Cup of Poison
ISBN 9781490860985

This book recounts the story I have been living for the past forty-five years. For many of those years, alcohol wrote my story for me. I was held captive by its addictive grip. My heart was closed to the greater purpose I was here to live. A tragedy helped open it, when I lost my niece to leukemia. Through all the trials, I came to know God and His meaning for my life as His child.

Endnotes

1   Available at https://www.goodreads.com/quotes/4432-until-one-has-loved-an-animal-a-part-of-one-s